THE
MEDITERRANEAN
DIET 2021

Recipes

51	Mediterranean Chicken with Pepperoncini and Kalamatas
52	Mediterranean Chicken and Bulgur Skillet
53	Chicken Florentine Soup
54	Roasted Chicken with Risotto and Caramelized Onions
55	Zucchini Pasta with Roasted Red Pepper Sauce and Chicken
56	Garlic Chicken Linguine
57	Fajita-Style Shrimp and Grits
58	Greek-Inspired Chicken Salad
59	Chicken Pesto Paninis
60	Swordfish with Olives, Capers & Tomatoes over Polenta
61	Orzo with Chicken and Artichokes
62	Chicken, Spinach, and Cheese Pasta Bake
63	Greek Lemon Chicken Soup
64	Zucchini Pasta
65	Greek Chicken Salad
66	Spanish Moroccan Fish
67	Mediterranean Power Lentil Salad
68	Chicken Breast Cutlets with Artichokes and Capers
69	Chakchouka(Shakshouka)
70	Mediterranean Cauliflower Pizza
71	Skillet Gnocchi with Chard & White Beans
72	Caramelized Onion, Olive & Anchovy Socca
73	Fasolakia(Greek Green Beans)

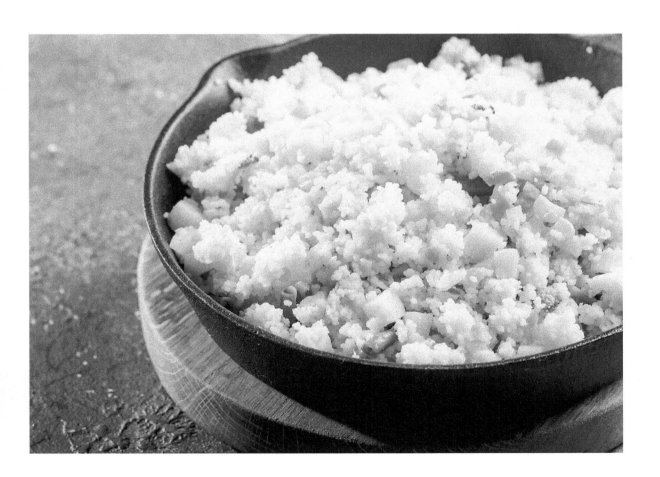

Mediterranean Cod with Roasted Tomatoes

PREPARATION
5 MIN

SERVES FOR
4 PEOPLE

INGREDIENTS

4 (4 ounce) fresh or frozen skinless cod fillets,
3/4- to 1-inch thick
2 teaspoons snipped fresh oregano
1 teaspoon snipped fresh thyme
1/2 teaspoon salt
1/4 teaspoon garlic powder
1/4 teaspoon paprika
1/4 teaspoon black pepper
Nonstick cooking spray
3 cups cherry tomatoes
2 cloves garlic, sliced
1 tablespoon olive oil
2 tablespoons sliced pitted ripe olives
2 teaspoons capers
Fresh oregano and/or thyme leaves

NUTRITION FACTS

Per Serving:
157 calories
protein 21.6g
carbohydrates 6.5g
fat 4.8g
cholesterol 48.8mg
sodium 429.2mg

STEPS

o Step
1. Preheat oven to 450 degrees F. Thaw fish, if frozen. Rinse fish and pat dry with paper towels. In a small bowl combine snipped oregano, snipped thyme, salt, garlic powder, paprika and black pepper. Sprinkle half of the oregano mixture over both sides of each fish fillet.
2. Line a 15x10x1-inch baking pan with foil. Coat foil with cooking spray. Place fish on one side of the foil-lined pan. Add tomatoes and garlic slices to the other side of the foil-lined pan. Combine remaining oregano mixture with oil. Drizzle oil mixture over tomatoes; toss to coat. Bake for 8 to 12 minutes or until fish flakes easily when tested with a fork, stirring tomato mixture once. Stir olives and capers into cooked tomato mixture.
3. Divide fish and roasted tomato mixture evenly among four serving plates. Garnish with fresh oregano and/or thyme leaves.

Linguine with Creamy White Clam Sauce

PREPARATION
15 MIN

SERVES FOR
4 PEOPLE

INGREDIENTS

8 ounces whole-wheat linguine
1 16-ounce container chopped clams (thawed if frozen) or two 10-ounce cans whole baby clams
3 tablespoons extra-virgin olive oil
3 cloves garlic, chopped
1/4 teaspoon crushed red pepper
1 tablespoon lemon juice
1/4 teaspoon salt
1 large tomato, chopped
1/4 cup chopped fresh basil, plus more for garnish
2 tablespoons heavy cream or half-and-half

NUTRITION FACTS

Per Serving:
421 calories
protein 21.5g
carbohydrates 51.9g
fat 16.6g
cholesterol 48.2mg
sodium 371.9mg

STEPS

o Step 1

1. Bring a large saucepan of water to a boil. Add pasta and cook until just tender, about 8 minutes or according to package directions. Drain.
2. Meanwhile, drain clams, reserving 3/4 cup of the liquid. Heat oil in a large skillet over medium-high heat. Add garlic and crushed red pepper and cook, stirring, for 30 seconds. Add the reserved clam liquid, lemon juice and salt; bring to a simmer and cook until slightly reduced, 2 to 3 minutes. Add tomato and the clams; bring to a simmer and cook for 1 minute more. Remove from heat.
3. Stir in basil and cream (or half-and-half). Add the pasta and toss to coat with the sauce. Garnish with more basil.

Fish Stew with Olives, Capers & Potatoes

PREPARATION
1 HOUR

SERVES FOR
4 PEOPLE

INGREDIENTS

1 1/4 pounds mahi-mahi, swordfish or halibut
steaks, about 3/4 inch thick
1/4 teaspoon sea salt
1/4 teaspoon ground pepper
6 canned plum tomatoes, drained and very
coarsely chopped
2 stalks celery, diced
1/2 medium red onion, halved and sliced
1 cup green olives, pitted
1/4 cup capers, preferably salt-packed, well
rinsed, plus more for garnish
1/4 cup extra-virgin olive oil
1 clove garlic, chopped
1/8 teaspoon crushed red pepper, or to taste
1 1/2 cups thinly sliced peeled yellow-fleshed
potatoes
1/4 cup chopped flat-leaf parsley

NUTRITION FACTS

Per Serving:

255 calories
protein 19.3g
carbohydrates 14.5g
fat 13.1g
cholesterol 69mg
sodium 314.9mg

STEPS

1. Pat fish dry and sprinkle both
    sides with salt and pepper. Set
    aside.
2. Combine tomatoes, celery, onion,
    olives, capers, oil, garlic and
    crushed red pepper in a large
    skillet and toss to mix well. Layer
    potato slices over the vegetables
    to cover them completely.
3. Cover the skillet and place over
    medium-low heat. Cook, adjusting
    the heat to keep a steady simmer
    and shaking the pan from time to
    time--but do not stir the vegeta-
    bles--until the potatoes are start-
    ing to soften, about 20 minutes.
4. Place the fish on top of the pota-
    toes, cover and continue cooking
    until the fish is opaque in the mid-
    dle, 10 to 12 minutes more. Serve
    sprinkled with parsley and more
    capers, if desired.

Salmon with Roasted Red Pepper Quinoa Salad

PREPARATION
15 MIN

SERVES FOR
4 PEOPLE

INGREDIENTS

3 tablespoons extra-virgin olive oil, divided
1 1/4 pounds skin-on salmon, preferably wild, cut into 4 portions
1/2 teaspoon salt, divided
1/2 teaspoon ground pepper, divided
2 tablespoons red-wine vinegar
1 clove garlic, grated
2 cups cooked quinoa
1 cup chopped roasted red bell peppers (from a 12-ounce jar), rinsed
1/4 cup chopped fresh cilantro
1/4 cup chopped toasted pistachios

STEPS

1. Heat 1 tablespoon oil in a large nonstick or cast-iron skillet over medium-high heat. Pat salmon dry and sprinkle the flesh with 1/4 teaspoon each salt and pepper. Add to the pan, skin-side up, and cook until lightly browned, 3 to 4 minutes. Turn and cook until it's just cooked through and flakes easily with a fork, 1 to 2 minutes more. Transfer to a plate.
2. Meanwhile, whisk the remaining 2 tablespoons oil, 1/4 teaspoon each salt and pepper, vinegar and garlic in a medium bowl. Add quinoa, peppers, cilantro and pistachios; toss to combine. Serve the salmon with the salad.

NUTRITION FACTS

Serving Size: About 1 1/4 Cups
Per Serving:

481 calories
protein 35.8g
carbohydrates 31g
fat 21g
cholesterol 66.3mg
sodium 707mg.

Beet & Shrimp Winter Salad

PREPARATION
15 MIN

SERVES FOR
1 PEOPLE

INGREDIENTS

Salad
2 cups lightly packed arugula
1 cup lightly packed watercress
1 cup cooked beet wedges
1/2 cup zucchini ribbons
1/2 cup thinly sliced fennel
1/2 cup cooked barley
4 ounces cooked, peeled shrimp, tails left on if desired
Fennel fronds for garnish
Vinaigrette
2 tablespoons extra-virgin olive oil
1 tablespoon red- or white-wine vinegar
1/2 teaspoon Dijon mustard
1/2 teaspoon minced shallot
1/4 teaspoon ground pepper
1/8 teaspoon salt

NUTRITION FACTS

Serving Size: 4 1/2 Cups Salad
Per Serving:

584 calories
protein 35g
carbohydrates 47g
fat 29.8g
cholesterol 214.3mg
sodium 653.6mg

STEPS

1. Arrange arugula, watercress, beets, zucchini, fennel, barley and shrimp on a large dinner plate.
2. Whisk oil, vinegar, mustard, shallot, pepper and salt in a small bowl, then drizzle over the salad. Garnish with fennel fronds, if desired.

Farfalle with Tuna, Lemon and Fennel

PREPARATION
5 MIN

SERVES FOR
4 PEOPLE

INGREDIENTS

6 ounces dried whole grain farfalle (bow-tie) pasta
1 (5 ounce) can solid white tuna (packed in oil)
1 Olive oil
1 cup fennel, thinly sliced (1 medium bulb)
2 cloves garlic, minced
1/2 teaspoon crushed red pepper
1/2 teaspoon salt
2 (14.5 ounce) cans no-salt-added diced tomatoes, undrained
2 tablespoons snipped fresh Italian (flat leaf) parsley
1 teaspoon lemon peel, finely shredded

NUTRITION FACTS

Serving Size: 1 1/4 Cups
Per Serving:

356 calories
protein 16.7g
carbohydrates 42.8g
fat 14.2g
cholesterol 11mg
sodium 380.1mg

STEPS

1. Cook pasta according to package directions, omitting salt; drain. Return pasta to pan; cover and keep warm. Meanwhile, drain tuna, reserving oil. If necessary, add enough olive oil to measure 3 tablespoons total.
2. In a medium saucepan heat the 3 tablespoons of reserved oil over medium heat. Add fennel; cook for 3 minutes, stirring occasionally. Add garlic, crushed red pepper and salt; cook and stir about 1 minute or just until garlic is golden.
3. Stir in tomatoes. Bring to boiling; reduce heat. Simmer, uncovered, for 5 to 6 minutes or until mixture starts to thicken. Stir in tuna; simmer, uncovered, about 1 minute more or until tuna is heated through.
4. Pour tuna mixture over pasta; stir gently to combine. Sprinkle each serving with parsley and lemon peel.

Creamy Salmon & Sugar Snap Cauliflower Gnocchi

PREPARATION
15 MIN

SERVES FOR
4 PEOPLE

INGREDIENTS

3 cups sugar snap peas (about 3/4 pound), trimmed
2 tablespoons water
1 (12 ounce) bag frozen cauliflower gnocchi
4 tablespoons cream cheese, cubed
2 tablespoons low-fat plain Greek yogurt
4 ounces flaked smoked salmon
Freshly ground pepper to taste

STEPS

1. Place peas in a microwave-safe bowl or baking dish and add water. Cover tightly and microwave on High until tender, about 2 minutes.
2. Cook gnocchi according to package directions.
3. Heat cream cheese in a nonstick skillet just until melted. Add the gnocchi, peas and yogurt. Stir to coat. Top with salmon and a sprinkle of pepper.

NUTRITION FACTS

Serving Size:1 Cup
Per Serving:

194 calories
protein 9.3g
carbohydrates 18g
fat 8.3g
cholesterol 21.9mg
sodium 240.6mg

Seared Salmon with Pesto Fettuccine

PREPARATION
20 MIN

SERVES FOR
4 PEOPLE

INGREDIENTS

8 ounces whole-wheat fettuccine
2/3 cup pesto
1 1/4 pounds wild salmon, skinned and cut into 4 portions
1/4 teaspoon salt
1/4 teaspoon ground pepper
1 tablespoon extra-virgin olive oil

STEPS

1. Bring a large pot of water to a boil. Add fettuccine and cook until just tender, about 9 minutes. Drain and transfer to a large bowl. Toss with pesto.
2. Meanwhile, season salmon with salt and pepper. Heat oil in a large cast-iron or nonstick skillet over medium-high heat. Add salmon and cook, turning once, until just opaque in the middle, 2 to 4 minutes per side. Serve the salmon with the pasta.

NUTRITION FACTS

Per Serving:

603 calories
protein 44g
carbohydrates 45.3g
fat 28.4g
cholesterol 79.6mg
sodium 537.1mg

Spaghetti with Halibut & Lemon

PREPARATION
1 HR 15 MIN

SERVES FOR
6 PEOPLE

INGREDIENTS

12 ounces halibut, skinned and cut in 1/2-inch cubes
6 tablespoons lemon juice
1/4 cup extra-virgin olive oil
3 tablespoons finely chopped red onion
2 tablespoons finely chopped flat-leaf parsley
1/4 teaspoon crushed red pepper
1/2 teaspoon salt plus 1 tablespoon, divided
1 small Yukon Gold potato (about 2 ounces)
12 ounces spaghetti

NUTRITION FACTS

Serving Size: Generous 1 Cup
Per Serving:

368 calories
protein 18.9g
carbohydrates 46.1g
fat 11.4g
cholesterol 27.8mg
sodium 374.8mg

STEPS

1. Combine halibut, lemon juice, oil, onion, parsley and crushed red pepper in a large bowl. Season with 1/2 teaspoon salt and mix well. Let stand at room temperature, stirring occasionally, until the fish is opaque throughout, at least 1 hour and up to 2 hours.
2. Place potato in a large saucepan, cover with cold water and bring to a boil. Reduce heat to medium and cook until very tender, 12 to 15 minutes. Remove the potato; peel when it's cool enough to handle. Keep the potato-cooking water and add enough water to the pot to make about 2 quarts total for cooking the pasta.
3. When the fish is done marinating, return the water to a boil. Add the remaining 1 tablespoon salt, then stir in pasta until all the strands are submerged. Cook according to package instructions until just tender.
4. Meanwhile, mash the potato through a ricer or with a fork. Add to the bowl with the fish and stir until well combined.
5. When the pasta is done, drain well and toss with the fish mixture. Serve at once.

Fish Stew with Olives, Capers & Potatoes

PREPARATION
1 HR

SERVES FOR
4 PEOPLE

INGREDIENTS

1 1/4 pounds mahi-mahi, swordfish or halibut steaks, about 3/4 inch thick
1/4 teaspoon sea salt
1/4 teaspoon ground pepper
6 canned plum tomatoes, drained and very coarsely chopped
2 stalks celery, diced
1/2 medium red onion, halved and sliced
1 cup green olives, pitted
1/4 cup capers, preferably salt-packed, well rinsed, plus more for garnish
1/4 cup extra-virgin olive oil
1 clove garlic, chopped
1/4 teaspoon crushed red pepper, or to taste
1 1/2 cups thinly sliced peeled yellow-fleshed potatoes
1/4 cup chopped flat-leaf parsley

NUTRITION FACTS

**Serving Size: 4 Oz. Fish & 1 Cup Vegetables
Per Serving:**

255 calories
protein 19.3g
carbohydrates 14.5g
fat 13.1g
cholesterol 69mg
sodium 314.9mg

STEPS

1. Pat fish dry and sprinkle both sides with salt and pepper. Set aside.
2. Combine tomatoes, celery, onion, olives, capers, oil, garlic and crushed red pepper in a large skillet and toss to mix well. Layer potato slices over the vegetables to cover them completely.
3. Cover the skillet and place over medium-low heat. Cook, adjusting the heat to keep a steady simmer and shaking the pan from time to time--but do not stir the vegetables--until the potatoes are starting to soften, about 20 minutes.
4. Place the fish on top of the potatoes, cover and continue cooking until the fish is opaque in the middle, 10 to 12 minutes more. Serve sprinkled with parsley and more capers, if desired.

Quick Shrimp Puttanesca

PREPARATION
15 MIN

SERVES FOR
4 PEOPLE

INGREDIENTS

8 ounces refrigerated fresh linguine noodles, preferably whole-wheat
1 tablespoon extra-virgin olive oil
1 pound peeled and deveined large shrimp
1 (15 ounce) can no-salt-added tomato sauce
1 1/4 cups frozen quartered artichoke hearts, thawed (8 ounces)
1/4 cup chopped pitted Kalamata olives
1 tablespoon capers, rinsed
1/4 teaspoon salt

STEPS

1. Bring a large pot of water to a boil. Cook linguine according to package instructions. Drain.
2. Meanwhile, heat oil in a large skillet over high heat. Add shrimp in a single layer and cook, undisturbed, until browned on the bottom, 2 to 3 minutes. Stir in tomato sauce. Add artichoke hearts, olives, capers and salt; cook, stirring often, until the shrimp is cooked through and the artichoke hearts are hot, 2 to 3 minutes longer.
3. Add the drained noodles to the sauce and stir to combine. Divide among 4 pasta bowls. Serve hot.

NUTRITION FACTS

Serving Size: 2 Cups
Per Serving:

390 calories
protein 36.7g
carbohydrates 43.4g
fat 8g
cholesterol 241mg
sodium 629mg

Shrimp Oreganata Cauliflower Gnocchi

PREPARATION
15 MIN

SERVES FOR
4 PEOPLE

INGREDIENTS

1 (12 ounce) bag frozen cauliflower gnocchi
1 pint grape tomatoes, halved
1 tablespoon olive oil
2 teaspoons minced garlic
1/4 teaspoon oregano
Pinch of salt
1 pound cooked peeled shrimp (31-40 per pound; thawed if frozen)

STEPS

1. Cook gnocchi according to package directions.
2. Combine tomatoes, oil, garlic, oregano and salt in a large microwave-safe bowl. Microwave on High until softened, about 1 minute. Stir in the gnocchi and shrimp.

NUTRITION FACTS

Serving Size: 1 Cup

Per Serving:

133 calories
protein 2g
carbohydrates 16.8g
fat 5.5g
sodium 40.3mg

Creamy Scallop & Pea Fettuccine

PREPARATION
40 MIN

SERVES FOR
5 PEOPLE

INGREDIENTS

8 ounces whole-wheat fettuccine
1 pound large dry sea scallops,
1/4 teaspoon salt, divided
1 tablespoon extra-virgin olive oil
1 8-ounce bottle clam juice,
1 cup low-fat milk
3 tablespoons all-purpose flour
1/4 teaspoon ground white pepper
3 cups frozen peas, thawed
3/4 cup finely shredded Romano cheese, divided
1/3 cup chopped fresh chives
1/2 teaspoon freshly grated lemon zest
1 teaspoon lemon juice

NUTRITION FACTS

Serving Size: 1 1/2 Cups
Per Serving:

413 calories
protein 29.5g;
carbohydrates 55.2g
fat 9.4g
cholesterol 38.6mg
sodium 938mg

STEPS

1. Bring a large pot of water to a boil. Cook fettuccine until just tender, 8 to 10 minutes or according to package instructions. Drain.
2. Meanwhile, pat scallops dry and sprinkle with 1/8 teaspoon salt. Heat oil in a large nonstick skillet over medium-high heat. Add the scallops and cook until golden brown, 2 to 3 minutes per side. Transfer to a plate.
3. Add clam juice to the pan. Whisk milk, flour, white pepper and the remaining 1/8 teaspoon salt in a medium bowl until smooth. Whisk the milk mixture into the clam juice. Bring the mixture to a simmer, stirring constantly. Continue stirring until thickened, 1 to 2 minutes. Return the scallops and any accumulated juices to the pan along with peas and return to a simmer. Stir in the fettuccine, 1/2 cup Romano cheese, chives, lemon zest and juice until combined. Serve with the remaining cheese sprinkled on top.

Sheet-Pan Shrimp & Beets

PREPARATION
15 MIN

SERVES FOR
4 PEOPLE

INGREDIENTS

1 pound small beets, peeled and cut into 1/2-inch pieces
2 tablespoons extra-virgin olive oil, divided
3/4 teaspoon salt, divided
3/4 teaspoon ground pepper, divided
6 cups chopped kale
1 1/4 pounds extra-large raw shrimp (16-20 count), peeled and deveined
1/2 teaspoon dry mustard
1/2 teaspoon dried tarragon
3 tablespoons unsalted sunflower seeds, toasted

STEPS

1. Preheat oven to 425 degrees F.
2. Toss beets with 1 tablespoon oil and 1/4 teaspoon each salt and pepper in a large bowl. Spread evenly on a rimmed baking sheet. Roast for 15 minutes.
3. Toss kale with the remaining 1 tablespoon oil and 1/4 teaspoon each salt and pepper in the bowl. Stir into the beets on the baking sheet.
4. Sprinkle shrimp with mustard, tarragon and the remaining 1/4 teaspoon each salt and pepper. Place on top of the vegetables. Roast until the shrimp are cooked and the vegetables are tender, 10 to 15 minutes more.
5. Transfer the shrimp to a serving platter. Stir sunflower seeds into the vegetables and serve with the shrimp.

NUTRITION FACTS

Serving Size: 1 Cup Vegetables & 4 Oz. Shrimp
Per Serving:

266 calories
protein 28.9g
carbohydrates 14.8g
fat 11.1g
cholesterol 198.6mg
sodium 680.7mg

Salmon & Asparagus with Lemon-Garlic Butter Sauce

PREPARATION
10 MIN

SERVES FOR
4 PEOPLE

INGREDIENTS

1 pound center-cut salmon fillet, preferably wild, cut into 4 portions
1 pound fresh asparagus, trimmed
1/2 teaspoon salt
1/2 teaspoon ground pepper
3 tablespoons butter
1 tablespoon extra-virgin olive oil
1/2 tablespoon grated garlic
1 teaspoon grated lemon zest
1 tablespoon lemon juice

STEPS

1. Preheat oven to 375 degrees F. Coat a large rimmed baking sheet with cooking spray.
2. Place salmon on one side of the prepared baking sheet and asparagus on the other. Sprinkle the salmon and asparagus with salt and pepper.
3. Heat butter, oil, garlic, lemon zest and lemon juice in a small skillet over medium heat until the butter is melted. Drizzle the butter mixture over the salmon and asparagus. Bake until the salmon is cooked through and the asparagus is just tender, 12 to 15 minutes.

NUTRITION FACTS

Serving Size: 1 Piece Salmon & About 5
    Spears Asparagus
Per Serving:

270 calories
protein 25.4g
carbohydrates 5.6g
fat 16.5g
cholesterol 75.9mg
sodium 350.5mg

Seafood Couscous Paella

PREPARATION
35 MIN

SERVES FOR
2 PEOPLE

INGREDIENTS

2 teaspoons extra-virgin olive oil
1 medium onion, chopped
1 clove garlic, minced
1/2 teaspoon dried thyme
1/2 teaspoon fennel seed
1/4 teaspoon salt
1/4 teaspoon freshly ground pepper
Pinch of crumbled saffron threads
1 cup no-salt-added diced tomatoes, with juice
1/4 cup vegetable broth
4 ounces bay scallops, tough muscle removed
4 ounces small shrimp, (41-50 per pound),
peeled and deveined
1/2 cup whole-wheat couscous

STEPS

1. Heat oil in a large saucepan over medium heat. Add onion; cook, stirring constantly, for 3 minutes. Add garlic, thyme, fennel seed, salt, pepper and saffron; cook for 20 seconds.
2. Stir in tomatoes and broth. Bring to a simmer. Cover, reduce heat and simmer for 2 minutes.
3. Increase heat to medium, stir in scallops and cook, stirring occasionally, for 2 minutes. Add shrimp and cook, stirring occasionally, for 2 minutes more. Stir in couscous. Cover, remove from heat and let stand for 5 minutes; fluff.

NUTRITION FACTS

Serving Size:1 1/2 Cups
Per Serving:

403 calories
protein 26.6g
carbohydrates 60.3g
fat 6.8g
cholesterol 104.5mg
sodium 1019.2mg

Scallop Piccata on Angel Hair

PREPARATION
35 MIN

SERVES FOR
4 PEOPLE

INGREDIENTS

1 pound dry sea scallops, tough muscle removed
1/4 teaspoon kosher salt
1/4 teaspoon freshly ground pepper
1 tablespoon extra-virgin olive oil
8 ounces whole-wheat angel hair pasta
1/2 cup white wine
1/2 cup clam juice
2 teaspoons cornstarch
1/4 cup chopped garlic
3 tablespoons lemon juice
1 tablespoon capers, rinsed and chopped
2 teaspoons butter
2 tablespoons chopped fresh parsley

NUTRITION FACTS

Serving Size:1 1/2 Cups
Per Serving:

370 calories
protein 22.8g
carbohydrates 52.1g
fat 6.9g
cholesterol 33.2mg
sodium 610mg

STEPS

1. Put a large pot of water on to boil.
2. Sprinkle scallops on both sides with salt and pepper. Heat oil in a large nonstick skillet over medium-high heat. Reduce heat to medium and add the scallops; cook, turning once, until browned on both sides, about 6 minutes total. Transfer to a plate.
3. Cook pasta in the boiling water until not quite tender, about 4 minutes. Drain and rinse.
4. Whisk wine, clam juice and cornstarch in a small bowl until smooth.
5. Cook garlic in the pan over medium-high heat, stirring often, until softened, 1 to 2 minutes. Add the wine mixture; bring to a boil and cook until thickened, about 2 minutes. Stir in lemon juice, capers and butter; cook until the butter melts, 1 to 2 minutes.
6. Return the scallops to the pan, add the pasta and cook, stirring gently, until heated through and coated with the sauce, about 1 minute. Stir in parsley and serve immediately.

Lemon-Caper Black Cod with Broccoli & Potatoes

PREPARATION
30 MIN

SERVES FOR
4 PEOPLE

INGREDIENTS

1 pound baby potatoes, halved
12 ounces precut broccoli florets
4 tablespoons extra-virgin olive oil, divided
1/2 teaspoon kosher salt, divided
1 pound skin-on black cod
1/2 teaspoon ground pepper
2 tablespoons capers, rinsed and patted dry
2 tablespoons lemon juice
1 tablespoon Dijon mustard
1 clove garlic, minced
1 tablespoon chopped fresh thyme or 1/4 teaspoon dried
3 tablespoons shredded Parmesan cheese

NUTRITION FACTS

**Serving Size: 3 Oz. Fish & About 1 Cup Vegetables
Per Serving:**

483 calories
protein 21.2g
carbohydrates 27.1g
fat 32.8g
cholesterol 58.3mg
sodium 389mg

STEPS

1. Preheat oven to 450degrees F. Coat a rimmed baking sheet with cooking spray.
2. Toss potatoes and broccoli with 1 tablespoon oil and 1/4 teaspoon salt in a large bowl. Transfer to the prepared baking sheet. Cook, stirring once, until tender, 20 to 25 minutes.
3. Meanwhile, pat cod dry and cut into 4 portions. Season with the remaining 1/4 teaspoon salt and pepper. Heat 1 tablespoon oil in a large nonstick skillet over medium heat. Add capers and cook until golden brown, 1 to 2 minutes. Using a slotted spoon, transfer the capers to a paper towel, leaving the oil in the pan. Place the cod skin-side down in the pan. Cook, undisturbed, for 5 minutes. Flip and cook until the fish flakes easily with a fork, 3 to 4 minutes more.
4. Combine the remaining 2 tablespoons oil, lemon juice, mustard and garlic in a small bowl.
5. Toss the potatoes and broccoli with thyme. Serve the vegetables and cod drizzled with the lemon vinaigrette and garnished with the capers and Parmesan.

Dijon Salmon with Green Bean Pilaf

PREPARATION
30 MIN

SERVES FOR
4 PEOPLE

INGREDIENTS

1 1/4 pounds wild salmon, skinned and cut into 4 portions
3 tablespoons extra-virgin olive oil, divided
1 tablespoon minced garlic
3/4 teaspoon salt
2 tablespoons mayonnaise
2 teaspoons whole-grain mustard
1/2 teaspoon ground pepper, divided
12 ounces pretrimmed haricots verts or thin green beans, cut into thirds
1 small lemon, zested and cut into 4 wedges
2 tablespoons pine nuts
1 8-ounce package precooked brown rice
2 tablespoons water
Chopped fresh parsley for garnish

NUTRITION FACTS

**Serving Size: 4 Oz. Fish & 1 Cup Pilaf
Per Serving:**

442 calories
protein 32.2g
carbohydrates 21.6g
fat 24.8g
cholesterol 69.2mg
sodium 605.2mg

STEPS

1. Preheat oven to 425 degrees F. Line a rimmed baking sheet with foil or parchment paper.
2. Brush salmon with 1 tablespoon oil and place on the prepared baking sheet. Mash garlic and salt into a paste with the side of a chef's knife or a fork. Combine a scant 1 teaspoon of the garlic paste in a small bowl with mayonnaise, mustard and 1/4 teaspoon pepper. Spread the mixture on top of the fish.
3. Roast the salmon until it flakes easily with a fork in the thickest part, 6 to 8 minutes per inch of thickness.
4. Meanwhile, heat the remaining 2 tablespoons oil in a large skillet over medium-high heat. Add green beans, lemon zest, pine nuts, the remaining garlic paste and 1/4 teaspoon pepper; cook, stirring, until the beans are just tender, 2 to 4 minutes. Reduce heat to medium. Add rice and water and cook, stirring, until hot, 2 to 3 minutes more.
5. Sprinkle the salmon with parsley, if desired, and serve with the green bean pilaf and lemon wedges.

Shrimp Piccata with Zucchini Noodles

PREPARATION
35 MIN

SERVES FOR
4 PEOPLE

INGREDIENTS

5-6 medium zucchini (2 1/4-2 1/2 pounds), trimmed
1/2 teaspoon salt
2 tablespoons butter
2 tablespoons extra-virgin olive oil, divided
2 cloves garlic, minced
1 pound raw shrimp, peeled and deveined, tails left on if desired
1 cup low-sodium chicken broth
1 tablespoon cornstarch
1/3 cup white wine
1/4 cup lemon juice
3 tablespoons capers, rinsed
2 tablespoons chopped fresh parsley

NUTRITION FACTS

Serving Size: 1 Cup Zucchini & About 3/4 Cup Sauce
Per Serving:

281 calories
protein 24.4g
carbohydrates 12.7g
fat 14.5g
cholesterol 174.1mg
sodium 516mg

STEPS

1. Using a spiral vegetable slicer or a vegetable peeler, cut zucchini lengthwise into long, thin strands or strips. Stop when you reach the seeds in the middle (seeds make the noodles fall apart). Place the zucchini "noodles" in a colander and toss with salt. Let drain for 15 to 30 minutes, then gently squeeze to remove any excess water.

2. Meanwhile, heat butter and 1 tablespoon oil in a large skillet over medium-high heat. Add garlic and cook, stirring, for 30 seconds. Add shrimp and cook, stirring, for 1 minute.

3. Whisk broth and cornstarch in a small bowl. Add to the shrimp along with wine, lemon juice and capers. Simmer, stirring occasionally, until the shrimp is just cooked through, 4 to 5 minutes. Remove from heat.

4. Heat the remaining 1 tablespoon oil in a large nonstick skillet over medium-high heat. Add the zucchini noodles and gently toss until hot, about 3 minutes. Serve the shrimp and sauce over the zucchini noodles, sprinkled with parsley.

Roasted Cod with Warm Tomato-Olive-Caper Tapenade

PREPARATION
25 MIN

SERVES FOR
4 PEOPLE

INGREDIENTS

1 pound cod fillet
3 teaspoons extra-virgin olive oil, divided
1/4 teaspoon freshly ground pepper
1 tablespoon minced shallot
1 cup halved cherry tomatoes
1/4 cup chopped cured olives
1 tablespoon capers, rinsed and chopped
1 1/2 teaspoons chopped fresh oregano
1 teaspoon balsamic vinegar

NUTRITION FACTS

**Serving Size: 3 Oz. Portion Cod & 1/4 Cup
  Sauce
Per Serving:**

151 calories
protein 15.4g
carbohydrates 3.9g
fat 8g
cholesterol 44.6mg
sodium 588.3mg

STEPS

1. Preheat oven to 450F. Coat a baking sheet with cooking spray.
2. Rub cod with 2 teaspoons oil. Sprinkle with pepper. Place on the prepared baking sheet. Transfer to the oven and roast until the fish flakes easily with a fork, 15 to 20 minutes, depending on the thickness of the fillet.
3. Meanwhile, heat the remaining 1 teaspoon oil in a small skillet over medium heat. Add shallot and cook, stirring, until beginning to soften, about 20 seconds. Add tomatoes and cook, stirring, until softened, about 112 minutes. Add olives and capers; cook, stirring, for 30 seconds more. Stir in oregano and vinegar; remove from heat. Spoon the tapenade over the cod to serve.

Greek Stuffed Portobello Mushrooms

PREPARATION
15 MIN

SERVES FOR
4 PEOPLE

INGREDIENTS

3 tablespoons extra-virgin olive oil, divided
1 clove garlic, minced
1/2 teaspoon ground pepper, divided
1/4 teaspoon salt
4 portobello mushrooms (about 14 ounces), wiped clean, stems and gills removed
1 cup chopped spinach
1/2 cup quartered cherry tomatoes
1/3 cup crumbled feta cheese
2 tablespoons pitted and sliced Kalamata olives
1 tablespoon chopped fresh oregano

STEPS

1. Preheat oven to 400 degrees F.
2. Combine 2 tablespoons oil, garlic, 1/4 teaspoon pepper and salt in a small bowl. Using a silicone brush, coat mushrooms all over with the oil mixture. Place on a large rimmed baking sheet and bake until the mushrooms are mostly soft, 8 to 10 minutes.
3. Meanwhile, combine spinach, tomatoes, feta, olives, oregano and the remaining 1 tablespoon oil in a medium bowl. Once the mushrooms have softened, remove from the oven and fill with the spinach mixture. Bake until the tomatoes have wilted, about 10 minutes.

NUTRITION FACTS

Serving Size: 1 Stuffed Mushroom
Per Serving:

151 calories
protein 4.5g
carbohydrates 6.6g
fat 8.5g
cholesterol 11mg
sodium 390.4mg

Mediterranean Stuffed Chicken Breasts

PREPARATION
25 MIN

SERVES FOR
8 PEOPLE

INGREDIENTS

1/2 cup crumbled feta cheese
1/2 cup chopped roasted red bell peppers
1/2 cup chopped fresh spinach
1/4 cup Kalamata olives, pitted and quartered
1 tablespoon chopped fresh basil
1 tablespoon chopped fresh flat-leaf parsley
2 cloves garlic, minced
4 (8 ounce) boneless, skinless chicken breasts
1/4 teaspoon salt
1/2 teaspoon ground pepper
1 tablespoon extra-virgin olive oil
1 tablespoon lemon juice

NUTRITION FACTS

Serving Size: 1 /2 Breast
Per Serving:

179 calories
protein 24.4g
carbohydrates 1.9g
fat 7.4g
cholesterol 71mg
sodium 352mg

STEPS

1. Preheat oven to 400 degrees F. Combine feta, roasted red peppers, spinach, olives, basil, parsley and garlic in a medium bowl.
2. Using a small knife, cut a horizontal slit through the thickest portion of each chicken breast to form a pocket. Stuff each breast pocket with about 1/3 cup of the feta mixture; secure the pockets using wooden picks. Sprinkle the chicken evenly with salt and pepper.
3. Heat oil in a large oven-safe skillet over medium-high heat. Arrange the stuffed breasts, top-sides down, in the pan; cook until golden, about 2 minutes. Carefully flip the chicken; transfer the pan to the oven. Bake until an instant-read thermometer inserted in the thickest portion of the chicken registers 165 degrees F, 20 to 25 minutes. Drizzle the chicken evenly with lemon juice. Remove the wooden picks from the chicken before serving.

Herby Mediterranean Fish with Wilted Greens & Mushrooms

PREPARATION
25 MIN

SERVES FOR
4 PEOPLE

INGREDIENTS

3 tablespoons olive oil, divided
1/2 large sweet onion, sliced
3 cups sliced cremini mushrooms
2 cloves garlic, sliced
4 cups chopped kale
1 medium tomato, diced
2 teaspoons Mediterranean Herb Mix, divided
1 tablespoon lemon juice
1/2 teaspoon salt, divided
1/2 teaspoon ground pepper, divided
4 (4 ounce) cod, sole, or tilapia fillets
Chopped fresh parsley, for garnish

NUTRITION FACTS

**Serving Size: 1 Piece Fish + 1/2 Cup
Vegetables
Per Serving:**

214 calories
protein 18g
carbohydrates 11g
fat 11g
cholesterol 45mg
sodium 598mg

STEPS

1. Heat 1 Tbsp. oil in a large sauce-pan over medium heat. Add onion; cook, stirring occasionally, until translucent, 3 to 4 minutes. Add mushrooms and garlic; cook, stirring occasionally, until the mushrooms release their liquid and begin to brown, 4 to 6 minutes. Add kale, tomato, and 1 tsp. herb mix. Cook, stirring occasionally, until the kale is wilted and the mushrooms are tender, 5 to 7 minutes. Stir in lemon juice and 1/4 tsp. each salt and pepper. Remove from heat, cover, and keep warm.
2. Sprinkle fish with the remaining 1 tsp. herb mix and 1/4 tsp. each salt and pepper. Heat the remaining 2 Tbsp. oil in a large nonstick skillet over medium-high heat. Add the fish and cook until the flesh is opaque, 2 to 4 minutes per side, depending on thickness. Transfer the fish to 4 plates or a serving platter. Top and surround the fish with the vegetables; sprinkle with parsley, if desired.

Cauliflower, Pancetta & Olive Spaghetti

PREPARATION
30 MIN

SERVES FOR
4 PEOPLE

INGREDIENTS

8 ounces whole-wheat spaghetti
1 tablespoon extra-virgin olive oil
4 cups finely chopped cauliflower
1/4 cup diced pancetta
2 cloves garlic, finely chopped
1/2 cup dry white wine
1/4 cup finely chopped roasted red peppers
8 pitted Kalamata olives, sliced
1 tablespoon butter
1/4 cup chopped flat-leaf parsley
1/4 teaspoon salt
1/4 teaspoon ground peppe

STEPS

1. Cook pasta for 1 minute less than the package directions. Reserve 1 cup pasta water, then drain.
2. Meanwhile, heat oil in a large skillet over medium heat. Cook cauliflower and pancetta, stirring occasionally, until the cauliflower is starting to brown, about 10 minutes. Add garlic and cook, stirring, for 30 seconds. Stir in wine, increase heat to high and cook, stirring occasionally, until almost evaporated, about 2 minutes. Stir in peppers, olives and butter. Add the pasta along with the reserved cooking water; simmer until the water is almost evaporated, 1 to 2 minutes more. Stir in parsley, salt and pepper.

NUTRITION FACTS

Serving Size:1 2/3 Cups
Per Serving:

372 calories
protein 12.2g
carbohydrates 51g
fat 12.4g
cholesterol 13.9mg
sodium 519.2mg

Seared Cod with Spinach-Lemon Sauce

PREPARATION
25 MIN

SERVES FOR
4 PEOPLE

INGREDIENTS

1 5-ounce package baby spinach
3 tablespoons water
1/2 cup lightly packed fresh parsley sprigs
4 teaspoons lemon juice
4 teaspoons orange juice
1 clove garlic, quartered
1/2 teaspoon salt, divided
1/2 teaspoon ground pepper, divided
1/4 teaspoon crushed red pepper
11/4 pounds cod , cut into 4 portions
1 tablespoon grapeseed oil or canola oil
1/4 cup sliced toasted almonds

NUTRITION FACTS

**Serving Size: 4 Oz. Fish & 2 Tbsp. Sauce
Per Serving:**

163 calories
protein 20.9g
carbohydrates 4.4g
fat 7g
cholesterol 55.8mg
sodium 393mg

STEPS

1. Place spinach and water in a microwave-safe bowl. Cover with plastic wrap and poke a few holes in it. Microwave on High until wilted, about 2 minutes.
2. Puree the wilted spinach (and any remaining water), parsley, lemon juice, orange juice, garlic, 1/4 teaspoon each salt and pepper and crushed red pepper in a blender until smooth. Set aside.
3. Sprinkle cod with the remaining 1/4 teaspoon each salt and pepper.
4. Heat oil in a large nonstick skillet over medium-high heat. Cook the cod, turning once, until golden brown and just cooked through, 5 to 7 minutes total. Transfer to a plate; tent with foil to keep warm.
5. Pour the reserved sauce into the pan and cook, stirring occasionally, until slightly thickened, about 1 minute. Serve the fish on top of the sauce, sprinkled with almonds.

Tomato-Pesto Socca

PREPARATION
1 HR

SERVES FOR
4 PEOPLE

INGREDIENTS

1 cup chickpea flour
1/2 teaspoon salt
1/4 teaspoon ground pepper
1 cup water
2 tablespoons extra-virgin olive oil, divided
1 medium plum tomato, thinly sliced
1/2 cup torn or shredded smoked fresh mozzarella
2 tablespoons fresh basil pesto

NUTRITION FACTS

Serving Size: 1 Slice Each
Per Serving:

236 calories
protein 9.8g
carbohydrates 14.8g
fat 15.3g
cholesterol 13.6mg
sodium 455.3mg

STEPS

1. Whisk flour, salt and pepper in a large bowl. Add water; whisk until smooth. Let rest while the oven preheats or refrigerate for up to 1 day.
2. Position racks in upper and lower thirds of oven. Place a 12-inch cast-iron skillet on the lower rack. Preheat to 450 degrees F for 30 minutes.
3. When the oven is preheated, carefully remove the hot pan and swirl in 1 tablespoon oil. Whisk the batter, pour it into the pan and swirl to coat. Top with tomato and mozzarella.
4. Bake until the bottom is browned and the edges are crispy, 16 to 20 minutes. Remove from the oven and, using a pastry brush, dab the socca with the remaining 1 tablespoon oil (brushing can dislodge the toppings).
5. Turn the broiler to high. Broil the socca on the upper rack until browned in spots, 1 to 3 minutes. Top with pesto and cut into wedges.

Provençal Baked Fish with Roasted Potatoes & Mushrooms

PREPARATION
15 MIN

SERVES FOR
4 PEOPLE

INGREDIENTS

1 pound Yukon Gold or red potatoes, cubed
1 pound mushrooms (shiitake, cremini, oyster or other fresh mushrooms), trimmed and sliced
2 tablespoons extra-virgin olive oil, divided
1/4 teaspoon salt
1/4 teaspoon ground pepper
2 cloves garlic, peeled and sliced
14 ounces halibut, grouper or cod fillet, cut into 4 portions
4 tablespoons lemon juice
1 teaspoon herbes de Provence
Fresh thyme for garnish

STEPS

1. Preheat oven to 425 degrees F.
2. Toss potatoes, mushrooms, 1 Tbsp. oil, salt, and pepper in a large bowl. Transfer to a 9x13-inch baking dish. Roast until the vegetables are just tender, 30 to 40 minutes.
3. Stir the vegetables, then stir in garlic. Place fish on top. Drizzle with lemon juice and the remaining 1 Tbsp. oil. Sprinkle with herbes de Provence. Bake until the fish is opaque in the center and flakes easily, 10 to 15 minutes. Garnish with thyme, if desired.

NUTRITION FACTS

Serving Size: 1 Fish Fillet + About 1/2 Cup Vegetables
Per Serving:

276 calories
protein 24.4g
carbohydrates 25.3g
fat 8.8g
cholesterol 48.6mg
sodium 218.9mg

Trapanese Pesto Pasta & Zoodles with Salmon

PREPARATION
35 MIN

SERVES FOR
6 PEOPLE

INGREDIENTS

2 zucchini (1 3/4 lbs. total)
1 teaspoon salt, divided
1/2 cup raw whole almonds, toasted
1 pound grape tomatoes (3 cups)
1 cup packed fresh basil leaves plus 1/4 cup chopped, divided
2-4 cloves garlic
1/4 teaspoon crushed red pepper
3 tablespoons olive oil, divided
8 ounces whole-wheat spaghetti
1 pound skinless salmon fillets (about 4 fillets), patted dry
1/4 teaspoon ground pepper, plus more for garnish
2 tablespoons grated Parmesan cheese

NUTRITION FACTS

Per Serving:

450 calories
protein 25.9g
carbohydrates 40.8g
fat 23.5g
cholesterol 41.6mg
sodium 459.1mg

STEPS

1. Bring a large pot of water to a boil. Cut zucchini into long thin strips with a spiralizer or vegetable peeler. Place in a colander set over a large bowl. Toss with 1/4 tsp. salt and let drain for 15 to 20 minutes.

2. Meanwhile, pulse almonds in a food processor until coarsely chopped. Add tomatoes, 1 cup basil leaves, garlic, and crushed red pepper; pulse until coarsely chopped. Add 2 Tbsp. oil and 1/2 tsp. salt and pulse until combined; set aside.

3. Cook spaghetti in the boiling water according to package directions. Drain and transfer to a large bowl. Gently squeeze the zucchini to remove excess water; add to the bowl with the spaghetti.

4. Heat the remaining 1 Tbsp. oil in a large skillet over medium-high heat until shimmering. Season salmon with pepper and the remaining 1/4 tsp. salt. Add the salmon to the pan; cook until the underside is golden and crispy, about 4 minutes. Transfer to a plate and use a fork to gently flake it apart.

5. Add the pesto to the spaghetti mixture; toss to coat. Gently stir in the salmon. Top with the remaining 1/4 cup chopped fresh basil. Garnish with Parmesan and additional pepper, if desired.

Mediterranean Shrimp and Pasta

PREPARATION
25 MIN

SERVES FOR
4 PEOPLE

INGREDIENTS

8 ounces fresh or frozen medium shrimp
Nonstick cooking spray
1 (14.5 ounce) can no-salt-added diced toma-toes, drained
1 cup sliced zucchini
1 large red sweet pepper, chopped (1 cup)
1/2 cup dry white wine or reduced-sodium chicken broth
2 cloves garlic, minced
8 pitted Kalamata olives, coarsely chopped
1/4 cup chopped fresh basil
1 tablespoon olive oil
1 1/2 teaspoons chopped fresh rosemary or 1/2 teaspoon dried rosemary, crushed
1/4 teaspoon salt
4 ounces dried acini di pepe or whole-wheat acini di pepe, cooked according to package directions
2 ounces reduced-fat feta cheese, crumbled

NUTRITION FACTS

**Serving Size: 3/4 Cup Shrimp Mixture And
   1/2 Cup Pasta
Per Serving:**

302 calories
protein 19.9g
carbohydrates 32.4g
fat 8g
cholesterol 90.3mg
sodium 571.5mg

STEPS

1. Thaw shrimp, if frozen. Peel and devein shrimp; cover and chill until ready to use. Lightly coat an unheated 1 1/2-quart slow cooker with cooking spray. In the slow cooker combine tomatoes, zucchini, sweet pepper, wine and garlic.
2. Cover and cook on low-heat setting for 4 hours or high-heat setting for 2 hours. (If no heat setting is available, cook for 3 hours.) Stir in the shrimp. If using low-heat setting, turn to high-heat setting. Cover and cook for 30 minutes more.
3. Stir in olives, basil, olive oil, rosemary and salt. Place cooked pasta in a serving bowl and top with shrimp mixture. Sprinkle feta cheese evenly over all.

Pita Melts

PREPARATION
20 MIN

SERVES FOR
6 PEOPLE

INGREDIENTS

1 (6 ounce) container plain low-fat yogurt
1/3 cup chopped, seeded cucumber
2 teaspoons snipped fresh mint or 1/2 teaspoon dried mint, crushed
1 clove garlic, minced
Dash salt
Nonstick cooking spray
3 large whole-wheat pita bread rounds, split in half horizontally
3 large plum tomatoes, thinly sliced crosswise
1/2 cup crumbled reduced-fat feta cheese (2 ounces)
1/4 (12 ounce) jar roasted red peppers

NUTRITION FACTS

Serving Size: 1/2 A Pita And 4 Meatballs
Per Serving:

266 calories
protein 26g
carbohydrates 26g
dietary fiber 4g
fat 7g
cholesterol 52mg
sodium 596mg

STEPS

1. In a small bowl, combine yogurt, cucumber, mint, garlic, and salt.
2. Preheat broiler. Line a very large baking sheet with foil; lightly coat foil with nonstick cooking spray. Place meatballs on the prepared pan. Broil 3 to 4 inches from the heat for 3 to 5 minutes or until heated through, turning once. Slide the foil and meatballs off the pan and onto a wire rack; cover meatballs with foil to keep warm.
3. Place pita bread halves, cut sides up, on the same baking sheet. Top pita halves with tomatoes, meatballs, and the feta cheese. Broil about 2 minutes or until heated through. Spoon yogurt mixture over pita melts. Top with the roasted red peppers.

Briam (Greek Baked Zucchini and Potatoes)

PREPARATION
30 MIN

SERVES FOR
4 PEOPLE

INGREDIENTS

2 pounds potatoes, peeled and thinly sliced
4 large zucchini, thinly sliced
4 small red onions, thinly sliced
6 ripe tomatoes, pureed
1/2 cup olive oil
2 tablespoons chopped fresh parsley
sea salt and freshly ground black pepper to taste

STEPS

1. Preheat oven to 400 degrees F (200 degrees C).
2. Spread potatoes, zucchini, and red onions in a 9x13-inch baking dish, or preferably a larger one. Use 2 baking dishes if necessary. Cover with pureed tomatoes, olive oil, parsley. Season with salt and freshly ground pepper. Toss all ingredients together so that the vegetables are evenly coated.
3. Bake in the preheated oven, stirring after 1 hour, until vegetables are tender and moisture has evaporated, about 90 minutes. Cool slightly before serving, or serve at room temperature.

NUTRITION FACTS

Per Serving:

534 calories
protein 11.3g
carbohydrates 65.8g
fat 28.3g
sodium 141.4mg

Mediterranean Zucchini and Chickpea Salad

PREPARATION
25 MIN

SERVES FOR
6 PEOPLE

INGREDIENTS

2 cups diced zucchini
1 (15 ounce) can chickpeas, drained and rinsed
1 cup halved grape tomatoes
3/4 cup chopped red bell pepper
1/2 cup chopped sweet onion
1/2 cup crumbled feta cheese
1/2 cup chopped Kalamata olives
1/3 cup olive oil
1/3 cup packed fresh basil leaves, roughly chopped
1/4 cup white balsamic vinegar
1 tablespoon chopped fresh rosemary
1 tablespoon capers, drained and chopped
1 clove garlic, minced
1/2 teaspoon dried Greek oregano
1 pinch crushed red pepper flakes
salt and ground black pepper to taste

STEPS

1. Mix zucchini, chickpeas, tomatoes, red bell pepper, onion, feta, Kalamata olives, olive oil, basil, vinegar, rosemary, capers, garlic, oregano, red pepper flakes, salt, and black pepper together in a large bowl.

NUTRITION FACTS

Per Serving:

258 calories
protein 5.6g
carbohydrates 19g
fat 18.5g
cholesterol 11.1mg
sodium 514.6mg

Grilled Mediterranean Salmon in Foil

PREPARATION
15 MIN

SERVES FOR
4 PEOPLE

INGREDIENTS

1 (10 ounce) basket cherry tomatoes, quartered
4 tablespoons extra-virgin olive oil
1 small shallot, finely chopped
2 tablespoons black olive tapenade
1/2 teaspoon salt
8 basil leaves
4 small fresh thyme sprigs
freshly ground black pepper to taste
4 (12x18-inch) pieces aluminum foil
4 (7 ounce) salmon filets, with skin

STEPS

1. Preheat an outdoor grill for high heat and lightly oil the grate. Close cover.
2. Combine cherry tomatoes, olive oil, shallot, tapenade, salt, basil, thyme, and pepper in a bowl; mix well.
3. Lay out foil on a work surface, shiny side-up. Place each salmon fillet skin side-down in the center of a piece of foil. Cover each piece of salmon with 1/4 of the cherry tomato mixture. Fold up the edges of the foil over the salmon to create a parcel, making sure to seal the edges well.
4. Turn down the heat of the grill and carefully place the foil parcels on the grate. Close the cover and cook until salmon is pale pink in the center and flakes easily with a fork, 7 to 8 minutes. Remove parcels and let them sit for a few minutes before opening.

NUTRITION FACTS

Per Serving:

493 calories
protein 36.2g
carbohydrates 9.5g
fat 34.4g
cholesterol 97.8mg
sodium 458.4mg

Air Fryer Potato Wedges

PREPARATION
5 MIN

SERVES FOR
4 PEOPLE

INGREDIENTS

2 medium Russet potatoes, cut into wedges
1 1/2 tablespoons olive oil
1/2 teaspoon paprika
1/2 teaspoon parsley flakes
1/2 teaspoon chili powder
1/2 teaspoon sea salt
1/8 teaspoon ground black pepper

STEPS

1. Preheat air fryer to 400 degrees F (200 degrees C).
2. Place potato wedges in a large bowl. Add olive oil, paprika, parsley, chili, salt, and pepper and mix well to combine.
3. Place 8 wedges in the basket of the air fryer and cook for 10 minutes.
4. Flip wedges with tongs and cook for an additional 5 minutes. Repeat with remaining 8 wedges.

NUTRITION FACTS

Per Serving:

129 calories
protein 2.3g
carbohydrates 19g
fat 5.3g
sodium 230.2mg

Mediterranean Chicken Sheet Pan Dinner

PREPARATION
15 MIN

SERVES FOR
4 PEOPLE

INGREDIENTS

1/4 cup extra-virgin olive oil
lemon, juiced
2 tablespoons balsamic vinegar
1 teaspoon dried tarragon
1 teaspoon dried oregano
1 teaspoon paprika
1 teaspoon salt
1/2 teaspoon black pepper
4 chicken thighs with skin
1 small red onion, sliced into petals
8 mini bell peppers, halved lengthwise and seeded
1 pound baby potatoes, halved
1 lemon, sliced
1/4 cup crumbled feta cheese
1/4 cup fresh parsley, chopped
8 pitted kalamata olives

NUTRITION FACTS

Per Serving:

533 calories
protein 23g
carbohydrates 41.3g
fat 32.4g
cholesterol 84.9mg
sodium 1112.8mg

STEPS

1. Preheat the oven to 425 degrees F (220 degrees C). Line a large rimmed baking sheet with aluminum foil.
2. Whisk olive oil, juice of 1 lemon, vinegar, tarragon, oregano, paprika, salt, and pepper together in a large bowl. Add chicken thighs, onion, baby bell peppers, and potatoes. Stir until everything is evenly coated.
3. Transfer vegetable-chicken mixture to the prepared baking sheet and spread in an even layer. Scatter lemon slices over the vegetables, making sure to leave the chicken uncovered so that the skin will brown.
4. Bake in preheated oven for about 40 minutes. Remove from oven and top with feta, parsley, and olives.

Creamy Italian White Bean Soup

PREPARATION
20 MIN

SERVES FOR
4 PEOPLE

INGREDIENTS

1 tablespoon vegetable oil
1 onion, chopped
1 stalk celery, chopped
1 clove garlic, minced
2 (16 ounce) cans white kidney beans, rinsed and drained
1 (14 ounce) can chicken broth
1/4 teaspoon ground black pepper
1/8 teaspoon dried thyme
2 cups water
1 bunch fresh spinach, rinsed and thinly sliced
1 tablespoon lemon juice

NUTRITION FACTS

Per Serving:

245 calories
protein 12g
carbohydrates 38.1g
fat 4.9g
cholesterol 2.4mg
sodium 1014.4mg

STEPS

1. In a large saucepan, heat oil. Cook onion and celery in oil for 5 to 8 minutes, or until tender. Add garlic, and cook for 30 seconds, continually stirring. Stir in beans, chicken broth, pepper, thyme and 2 cups water. Bring to a boil, reduce heat, and then simmer for 15 minutes.
2. With slotted spoon, remove 2 cups of the bean and vegetable mixture from soup and set aside.
3. In blender at low speed, blend remaining soup in small batches until smooth, (it helps to remove the center piece of the blender lid to allow steam to escape.) Once blended pour soup back into stock pot and stir in reserved beans.
4. Bring to a boil, occasionally stirring. Stir in spinach and cook 1 minute or until spinach is wilted. Stir in lemon juice and remove from heat and serve with fresh grated Parmesan cheese on top.

Slow Cooker Mediterranean Roast Turkey Breast

PREPARATION
20 MIN

SERVES FOR
8 PEOPLE

INGREDIENTS

1 (4 pound) boneless turkey breast, trimmed
1/2 cup chicken broth, divided
2 tablespoons fresh lemon juice
2 cups chopped onion
1/2 cup pitted kalamata olives
1/2 cup oil-packed sun dried tomatoes, thinly sliced
1 teaspoon Greek seasoning
1/2 teaspoon salt
1/4 teaspoon fresh ground black pepper
3 tablespoons all-purpose flour

STEPS

1. Place turkey breast, 1/4 cup chicken broth, lemon juice, onion, kalamata olives, sun-dried tomatoes, Greek seasoning, salt, and pepper in the crock of a slow cooker. Cover; cook on Low for 7 hours.
2. Combine the remaining 1/4 cup chicken broth and the flour in a small bowl; whisk until smooth. Stir into slow cooker. Cover and cook on Low for an additional 30 minutes.

NUTRITION FACTS

Per Serving:

333 calories
protein 60.6g
carbohydrates 8.9g
fat 4.7g
cholesterol 163.8mg
sodium 464.8mg

Slow Cooker Mediterranean Beef with Artichokes

PREPARATION
20 MIN

SERVES FOR
6 PEOPLE

INGREDIENTS

1 tablespoon grapeseed oil
2 pounds stewing beef
1 (14 ounce) can artichoke hearts, drained and halved
1 onion, diced
4 cloves garlic, chopped or more to taste
1 (32 fluid ounce) container beef broth
1 (15 ounce) can tomato sauce
1 (14.5 ounce) can diced tomatoes
1/2 cup pitted and roughly chopped Kalamata olives
1 teaspoon dried oregano
1 teaspoon dried parsley
1 teaspoon dried basil
1/2 teaspoon ground cumin
1 bay leaf

STEPS

1. Heat oil in a large pot over medium-high heat. Cook beef in the hot oil until browned, about 2 minutes per side.
2. Transfer beef to a slow cooker. Cover with artichoke hearts, onion, and garlic. Pour in beef broth, tomato sauce, and diced tomatoes. Stir in olives, oregano, parsley, basil, cumin, bay leaf.
3. Cook on Low until beef is tender, about 7 hours.

NUTRITION FACTS

Per Serving:

416 calories
protein 29.9g
carbohydrates 14.1g
fat 26.2g
cholesterol 83.5mg;
sodium 1452.8mg

Slow Cooker Chicken Marrakesh

PREPARATION
25 MIN

SERVES FOR
8 PEOPLE

INGREDIENTS

1 onion, sliced
2 cloves garlic, minced
2 large carrots, peeled and diced
2 large sweet potatoes, peeled and diced
1 (15 ounce) can garbanzo beans, drained and rinsed
2 pounds skinless, boneless chicken breast halves, cut into 2-inch pieces
1/2 teaspoon ground cumin
1/2 teaspoon ground turmeric
1/4 teaspoon ground cinnamon
1/2 teaspoon ground black pepper
1 teaspoon dried parsley
1 teaspoon salt
1 (14.5 ounce) can diced tomatoes

STEPS

1. Place the onion, garlic, carrots, sweet potatoes, garbanzo beans, and chicken breast pieces into a slow cooker. In a bowl, mix the cumin, turmeric, cinnamon, black pepper, parsley, and salt, and sprinkle over the chicken and vegetables. Pour in the tomatoes, and stir to combine.
2. Cover the cooker, set to High, and cook until the sweet potatoes are tender and the sauce has thickened, 4 to 5 hours.

NUTRITION FACTS

Per Serving:

290 calories
protein 30.6g
carbohydrates 36g
fat 2g
cholesterol 65.9mg
sodium 625mg

Easy Roasted Tomato Basil Soup

PREPARATION
10 MIN

SERVES FOR
6 PEOPLE

INGREDIENTS

3 lb Roma tomatoes halved
2 to 3 carrots peeled and cut into small chunks
Extra virgin olive oil
Salt and pepper
2 medium yellow onions chopped
5 garlic cloves minced
1 cup canned crushed tomatoes
2 oz fresh basil leaves
3 to 4 fresh thyme springs 2 tsp thyme leaves
1 tsp dry oregano
1/2 tsp paprika
1/2 tsp ground cumin
2 1/2 cups water
Splash of lime juice optional

NUTRITION FACTS

Per Serving:

Calories: 104.9kcal
Carbohydrates: 23.4g
Protein: 4.3g
Fat: 0.8g
Saturated Fat: 0.1g
Fiber: 5.4g
Sugar: 14.3g

STEPS

o Step
1. Heat oven to 450 degrees F.
2. In a large mixing bowl, combine tomatoes and carrot pieces. Add a generous drizzle of extra virgin olive oil, and season with kosher salt and black pepper. Toss to combine.
3. Transfer to a large baking sheet and spread well in one layer. Roast in heated oven for about 30 minutes. When ready, remove from the heat and set aside for about 10 minutes to cool.
4. Transfer the roasted tomatoes and carrots to the large bowl of a food processor fitted with a blade. Add just a tiny bit of water and blend.
5. In a large cooking pot, heat 2 tbsp extra virgin olive oil over medium-high heat until shimmering but not smoking. Add onions and cook for about 3 minutes, then add garlic and cook briefly until golden.
6. Pour the roasted tomato mixture into the cooking pot. Stir in crushed tomatoes, 2 1/2 cups water, basil, thyme and spices. Season with a little kosher salt and black pepper. Bring to a boil, then lower heat and cover part-

way. Let simmer for about 20 minutes or so.

Remove the thyme springs and transfer tomato basil soup to serving bowls. If you like, add a splash of lime juice and a generous drizzle of extra virgin olive oil. Serve with your favorite crusty bread or grilled pieces of French baguette.

Slow Cooker Spanish Beef Stew

PREPARATION
10 MIN

SERVES FOR
6 PEOPLE

INGREDIENTS

1 pound beef stew meat
salt and ground black pepper to taste
1/2 cup chopped Spanish onion
2 cloves garlic, minced
2 cups chopped red potatoes
1 (14.5 ounce) can diced tomatoes
1 (12 ounce) jar sofrito
1/2 cup pitted and halved green olives

STEPS

1. Heat a large skillet over medium heat. Cook beef in hot skillet until completely browned, about 5 minutes; season with salt and pepper. Transfer beef to a slow cooker, retaining some of the beef drippings in the skillet.
2. Return skillet to heat and heat the retained drippings. Saute onion and garlic in hot drippings until softened, about 5 minutes; add to beef in slow cooker.
3. Stir potatoes, diced tomatoes, sofrito, and olives into the beef mixture.
4. Cook on Low until beef and potatoes are fork-tender, 4 to 5 hours.

NUTRITION FACTS

Per Serving:

241 calories
protein 19.6g
carbohydrates 13.6g
fat 11.6g
cholesterol 39.8mg
sodium 821.7mg

Mediterranean Chicken with Pepperoncini and Kalamatas

PREPARATION
20 MIN

SERVES FOR
4 PEOPLE

INGREDIENTS

12 pepperoncini peppers, rinsed and drained
1 cup sliced pitted kalamata olives
8 cloves minced garlic
3 1/2 pounds chicken leg quarters
1 1/2 teaspoons paprika
1/4 teaspoon salt
1/4 teaspoon fresh ground pepper
1/2 teaspoon grated lemon zest
1/2 cup fresh-squeezed lemon juice
1 cup sour cream
1/2 teaspoon paprika

NUTRITION FACTS

Per Serving:

841 calories
protein 68.1g
carbohydrates 13.8g
fat 55.9g
cholesterol 248.7mg
sodium 2694.3mg

STEPS

1. Layer whole pepperoncini on the bottom of a slow cooker. Sprinkle the olive slices and garlic on top of the peppers.
2. Rinse chicken and pat dry. Place on top of pepperoncini mixture. Sprinkle chicken with 1 1/2 teaspoons paprika, the salt, pepper and lemon zest. Slowly pour in lemon juice.
3. Cover and cook on low 6 to 6 1/2 hours or until meat easily pulls away from bone. Remove chicken to a warm plate and cover to keep warm.
4. Turn slow cooker on high. Skim fat from cooking liquid. Whisk in sour cream until blended. Cover and simmer on high until heated through 8 to 10 minutes depending on your cooker. Stir in pepper and paprika.

Mediterranean Chicken and Bulgur Skillet

PREPARATION
25 MIN

SERVES FOR
4 PEOPLE

INGREDIENTS

4 (6-oz.) skinless, boneless chicken breasts
3/4 teaspoon kosher salt, divided
1/2 teaspoon freshly ground black pepper, divided
1 tablespoon olive oil, divided
1 cup thinly sliced red onion
1 tablespoon thinly sliced garlic
1/2 cup uncooked bulgur
2 teaspoons chopped fresh or 1/2 tsp. dried oregano
4 cups chopped fresh kale (about 2 1/2 oz.)
1/2 cup thinly sliced bottled roasted red bell peppers
1 cup unsalted chicken stock
2 ounces feta cheese, crumbled (about 1/2 cup)
1 tablespoon coarsely chopped fresh dill

NUTRITION FACTS

Per Serving:

Calories 369
Fat 11.3g
Carbohydrate 21g
Cholesterol 137mg
Sodium 663mg

STEPS

1. Preheat oven to 400 F.
2. Sprinkle chicken with 1/2 teaspoon salt and 1/4 teaspoon black pepper. Heat 1 1/2 teaspoons oil in a 10-inch cast-iron or other ovenproof skillet over medium-high. Add chicken to pan; cook until browned on both sides, about 3 minutes per side. Transfer chicken to a plate.
3. Add remaining oil to pan. Add onion and garlic; cook, stirring occasionally, until lightly browned, about 5 minutes. Add bulgur and oregano; cook, stirring often, until fragrant and toasted, about 2 minutes. Add kale and bell peppers; cook, stirring constantly, until kale begins to wilt, about 2 minutes. Add stock and remaining 1/4 teaspoon each salt and black pepper; bring to a boil. Remove from heat.
4. Nestle chicken into bulgur mixture; place skillet in oven. Bake at 400F until a meat thermometer inserted in thickest portion of chicken registers 165F, 12 to 15 minutes. Remove from oven. Sprinkle with feta. Let stand 5 minutes. Sprinkle with dill, and serve immediately.

Chicken Florentine Soup

PREPARATION
20 MIN

SERVES FOR
4 PEOPLE

INGREDIENTS

2 tablespoons olive oil
1 onion, chopped
1 cup diced carrots
1 cup diced celery
2 cloves garlic, minced
1 cup baby spinach leaves
4 cups 99% fat-free chicken broth
1 (15 ounce) can diced tomatoes
1 lemon, juiced
1/4 teaspoon ground black pepper
1/4 teaspoon dried oregano
1/4 teaspoon dried sweet basil
2 cups diced cooked chicken
1 cup cooked white rice

STEPS

1. Heat olive oil in a large pot over medium heat. Add onion, carrots, celery, and garlic; cook and stir until onion is translucent, about 5 minutes. Stir in baby spinach.
2. Pour chicken broth, diced tomatoes, and lemon juice into the pot. Stir in pepper, oregano, and basil. Bring to a boil; stir in chicken and rice. Reduce heat to medium-low and simmer until flavors combine, about 30 minutes.

NUTRITION FACTS

Per Serving:

350 calories
protein 21.9g
carbohydrates 26g
fat 16.5g
cholesterol 60.5mg
sodium 1408.4mg

Roasted Chicken with Risotto and Caramelized Onions

PREPARATION
15 MIN

SERVES FOR
4 PEOPLE

INGREDIENTS

4 tablespoons olive oil, divided
1 onion, chopped
1/4 cup balsamic vinegar
1 1/2 cups uncooked Arborio rice
1/4 cup dry white wine
7 cups hot chicken broth
2 tablespoons butter
2 cups chopped cooked chicken breast
salt and pepper to taste
2 tablespoons chopped fresh thyme

NUTRITION FACTS

Per Serving:

774 calories
protein 44.8g
carbohydrates 77.3g
fat 29.1g
cholesterol 72.2mg
sodium 2840.1mg

STEPS

1. Heat 2 tablespoons of the oil in a medium saucepan over medium heat. Stir in the onions and saute for 15 to 20 minutes, or until the onions are a dark golden brown. Remove from heat, stir in the balsamic vinegar and set aside.

2. Heat the remaining oil in a separate large skillet over medium heat. Stir in the rice and mix well. Let heat for about 2 minutes, then pour in the wine. Reduce heat to medium low and start pouring in the broth about 1 cup at a time. Add more broth as each cup is absorbed. Continue in this manner until all the broth is absorbed and the rice is al dente, about 20 minutes.

3. Stir in the reserved onion mixture and allow to heat through. Remove from heat and stir in the butter and chicken. Season with salt and pepper to taste, and garnish each serving with fresh thyme.

Zucchini Pasta with Roasted Red Pepper Sauce and Chicken

PREPARATION
1 HOUR

SERVES FOR
4 PEOPLE

INGREDIENTS

6 roma tomatoes
3 red bell peppers, chopped
1 large sweet onion, halved
3 tablespoons extra-virgin olive oil
4 cloves garlic
1 (28 ounce) can crushed tomatoes
1 cup tightly packed fresh basil leaves, chopped
salt and ground black pepper to taste
2 yellow summer squash, cut into spirals using a spiral slicer
2 zucchini, cut into spirals using a spiral slicer
2 cooked chicken breast halves, cubed
1 tablespoon grated Parmesan cheese, or to taste

NUTRITION FACTS

Per Serving:

352 calories
protein 23.3g
carbohydrates 33.4g
fat 16g
cholesterol 42.3mg
sodium 369.2mg

STEPS

1. Preheat grill for medium heat and lightly oil the grate.
2. Grill tomatoes, bell peppers, and onion halves on the preheated grill until well charred, about 15 minutes. When peppers are cool enough to handle, split with a knife and remove seeds.
3. Heat olive oil in a large skillet; cook and stir garlic until fragrant, about 1 minute. Stir canned crushed tomatoes, basil, grilled tomatoes, bell peppers, and onion into skillet; bring to a boil, reduce heat, and simmer until vegetables are tender, about 10 minutes. Puree vegetable mixture with a stick blender; season with salt and pepper and keep at a simmer.
4. Bring a large pot of water to a boil; drop in summer squash and zucchini spirals and cook until tender, about 3 minutes. Drain water from pot; lay spirals on paper towels to drain completely.
5. Place squash spirals on individual plates; top with a portion of cooked chicken, a generous amount of red pepper sauce, and Parmesan cheese.

Garlic Chicken Linguine

PREPARATION
20 MIN

SERVES FOR
8 PEOPLE

INGREDIENTS

1 (16 ounce) package linguine pasta
1/4 cup olive oil
1/4 cup chopped garlic
6 tomatoes, skinned and chopped, or more to taste
4 cups chopped cooked chicken
10 slices prosciutto, cut into small pieces, or more to taste
1/4 cup chopped fresh basil, or to taste
1/4 cup grated Romano cheese

STEPS

1. Bring a large pot of lightly salted water to a boil. Cook linguine at a boil until tender yet firm to the bite, about 11 minutes; drain and transfer to a serving bowl.
2. Combine olive oil and garlic in a saucepan over medium heat; cook and stir until fragrant, about 3 minutes. Add tomatoes; cover saucepan and simmer until tomatoes are cooked down into a sauce, 7 to 10 minutes.
3. Mix chicken, prosciutto, and basil into tomato sauce; cook and stir until chicken is heated through, about 3 minutes. Spoon sauce over pasta and top with Romano cheese.

NUTRITION FACTS

Per Serving:

497 calories
protein 32.6g
carbohydrates 46.7g
fat 20.2g
cholesterol 72.2mg
sodium 445.2mg

Fajita-Style Shrimp and Grits

PREPARATION
30 MIN

SERVES FOR
4 PEOPLE

INGREDIENTS

1 pound uncooked shrimp (16-20 per pound),
peeled and deveined
2 tablespoons fajita seasoning mix
1 cup quick-cooking grits
4 cups boiling water
1-1/2 cups shredded Mexican cheese blend
3 tablespoons 2% milk
2 tablespoons canola oil
3 medium sweet peppers, seeded and cut into
1-inch strips
1 medium sweet onion, cut into 1-inch strips
1 jar (15-1/2 to 16 ounces) chunky medium salsa
1/4 cup orange juice
1/4 cup plus 1 tablespoon fresh cilantro leaves,
divided

STEPS

1. Sprinkle shrimp with fajita seasoning; toss to coat. Set aside.
2. Slowly stir grits into boiling water. Reduce heat to medium; cook, covered, stirring occasionally, until thickened, 5-7 minutes. Remove from heat. Stir in cheese until melted; stir in milk. Keep warm.
3. In a large skillet, heat oil over medium-high heat. Add peppers and onion; cook and stir until tender and pepper edges are slightly charred. Add salsa, orange juice and shrimp. Cook, stirring constantly, until shrimp turn pink, 4-6 minutes. Stir in 1/4 cup cilantro. Remove from heat.
4. Spoon grits into serving bowls; top with shrimp mixture. Sprinkle with remaining cilantro.

NUTRITION FACTS

Per Serving:

561 calories
protein 33g
carbohydrates 55g
fat 23g
cholesterol 176mg
sodium 1324mg

Greek-Inspired Chicken Salad

PREPARATION
30 MIN

SERVES FOR
4 PEOPLE

INGREDIENTS

1 cup diced English cucumbers
1 1/4 teaspoons salt, divided
2 tablespoons diced red onion
1 cup Greek yogurt
1/3 cup chopped Kalamata olives
1 1/2 tablespoons chopped fresh dill
2 teaspoons red wine vinegar
2 teaspoons lemon juice
1 teaspoon garlic, minced
1 teaspoon lemon zest
1/2 teaspoon dried oregano
1/4 teaspoon ground black pepper
3 cups diced cooked chicken
3/4 cup crumbled feta cheese
1/2 cup diced seeded plum tomatoes
1 head Bibb lettuce, or more as needed

NUTRITION FACTS

Per Serving:

385 calories
protein 37.1g
carbohydrates 8.7g
fat 22g
cholesterol 115mg
sodium 1326.7mg

STEPS

1. Place cucumbers in a colander; set onto a plate. Toss cucumbers with 1 teaspoon salt. Let rest to draw about liquid, about 30 minutes. Pat dry with paper towels.
2. Place red onion and 1 cup cold water in a bowl. Let soak until the strong onion flavor is weakened, 5 to 10 minutes. Drain and rinse.
3. Combine cucumbers, red onions, Greek yogurt, Kalamata olives, dill, vinegar, lemon juice, garlic, lemon zest, oregano, and black pepper in a bowl. Fold in chicken, feta cheese, and tomatoes. Cover with plastic wrap; refrigerate salad for at least 1 hour.
4. Stir salad and serve on lettuce leaves.

Chicken Pesto Paninis

PREPARATION
15 MIN

SERVES FOR
4 PEOPLE

INGREDIENTS

1 focaccia bread, quartered
1/2 cup prepared basil pesto
1 cup diced cooked chicken
1/2 cup diced green bell pepper
1/4 cup diced red onion
1 cup shredded Monterey Jack cheese

STEPS

1. Preheat a panini grill.
2. Slice each quarter of focaccia bread in half horizontally. Spread each half with pesto. Layer bottom halves with equal amounts chicken, bell pepper, onion, and cheese. Top with remaining focaccia halves, forming 4 sandwiches.
3. Grill paninis 5 minutes in the preheated grill, or until focaccia bread is golden brown and cheese is melted.

NUTRITION FACTS

Per Serving:

641 calories
protein 32.4g
carbohydrates 60.9g
fat 29.4g
cholesterol 61.4mg
sodium 1075.5mg

Swordfish with Olives, Capers & Tomatoes over Polenta

PREPARATION
20 MIN

SERVES FOR
4 PEOPLE

INGREDIENTS

2 1/2 cups water
1/2 teaspoon salt, divided
1/2 cup coarse or regular yellow cornmeal or polenta
1 tablespoon extra-virgin olive oil
4 medium stalks celery, diced
2 cloves garlic, minced
1 (15 ounce) can no-salt-added diced tomatoes
1/4 cup green olives, such as Sicilian colossal or Cerignola, rinsed, pitted and coarsely chopped
3 tablespoons chopped fresh basil
1 tablespoon capers, rinsed
1/8 teaspoon ground pepper
Pinch of crushed red pepper
1 pound swordfish, cut into 4 steaks
Fresh basil for garnish

NUTRITION FACTS

Per Serving:

276 calories
protein 22.1g
carbohydrates 18.9g
fat 12.1g
cholesterol 64.6mg
sodium 536.4mg

STEPS

1. Bring 2 cups water to a boil in a medium saucepan over high heat. Add 1/4 tsp. salt. Slowly pour in cornmeal in a gentle stream, stirring rapidly with a whisk. Cook, stirring, until the mixture starts to thicken, about 3 minutes.
2. Reduce heat to a low simmer. Cook, stirring every 5 minutes, until the polenta easily comes away from the sides of the pan, 20 to 25 minutes. While stirring, crush any lumps against the side of the pan. If the polenta becomes too thick to stir, add 1/2 cup water. Remove from heat and cover to keep warm.
3. Meanwhile, heat oil in a large skillet over medium heat. Add celery; cook, stirring occasionally, until tender, about 5 minutes. Add garlic; cook until aromatic but not browned, 30 seconds. Stir in tomatoes, olives, basil, capers, ground pepper, crushed red pepper, and the remaining 1/4 tsp. salt. Cover, reduce heat to low, and simmer for 5 minutes.
4. Place swordfish steaks in the simmering sauce. Cover and cook until the fish is cooked through, 10 to 15 minutes.
5. To serve, spoon the polenta onto a large serving platter. Arrange the fish over the polenta, top with the sauce, and garnish with fresh basil, if desired.

Orzo with Chicken and Artichokes

PREPARATION
20 MIN

SERVES FOR
4 PEOPLE

INGREDIENTS

3 teaspoons olive oil, divided
3 ounces pancetta bacon, diced
1/2 medium onion, chopped
1 clove garlic, minced
1/4 teaspoon crushed red pepper flakes
1/2 cup dry white wine
1 1/2 cups cubed, cooked chicken
1 (10 ounce) can artichoke hearts (water-packed), quartered
5 ounces baby spinach
1 (16 ounce) package orzo pasta
2 tablespoons pine nuts, toasted
1/8 cup balsamic vinegar

NUTRITION FACTS

Per Serving:

758 calories
protein 35.5g
carbohydrates 96.6g
fat 23.6g
cholesterol 55.2mg
sodium 678.6mg

STEPS

1. Heat 1 tablespoon olive oil in a large skillet over medium heat. Stir in pancetta, and cook until browned. Remove to paper towels.
2. Pour 2 tablespoons olive oil into skillet. Stir in onion, garlic, and red pepper flakes. Cook, stirring occasionally, until the onion is soft and translucent. Increase heat to medium high, pour in white wine; cook about 3 minutes.
3. Reduce heat to low, stir in chicken, artichoke hearts, and spinach. Cover, and cook to warm through.
4. Meanwhile, bring a pot of salted water to boil. Add orzo pasta and cook until al dente, about 8 to 10 minutes. Drain, and stir into chicken mixture.
5. Stir pine nuts and balsamic vinegar into pasta.

Chicken, Spinach, and Cheese Pasta Bake

PREPARATION
15 MIN

SERVES FOR
8 PEOPLE

INGREDIENTS

1 (8 ounce) package penne pasta
1 teaspoon olive oil
1 onion, chopped
3 cups chopped cooked chicken
1 (14 ounce) can Italian-style diced tomatoes
1 (10 ounce) package spinach
1 (8 ounce) package cream cheese, softened
1 1/2 cups shredded mozzarella cheese

STEPS

1. Preheat oven to 375 degrees F (190 degrees C).
2. Bring a large pot of lightly salted water to a boil; add penne and cook, stirring occasionally, until tender yet firm to the bite, about 11 minutes. Drain.
3. Heat olive oil in a skillet over medium-high heat. Saute onion in hot oil until tender, 5 to 7 minutes.
4. Mix penne pasta, onion, chicken, diced tomatoes, spinach, and cream cheese together in a baking dish until the cream cheese melts and coats everything. Sprinkle mozzarella cheese over the pasta mixture. Cover baking dish with aluminum foil.
5. Bake in the preheated oven for 30 minutes. Remove foil and continue baking until heated through and beginning to brown along the edges, about 15 minutes more.

NUTRITION FACTS

Per Serving:

544 calories
protein 34.2g
carbohydrates 53.2g
fat 21.7g
cholesterol 85.3mg
sodium 331.9mg

Greek Lemon Chicken Soup

PREPARATION
25 MIN

SERVES FOR
6 PEOPLE

INGREDIENTS

8 cups chicken broth
1/2 cup fresh lemon juice
1/2 cup shredded carrots
1/2 cup chopped onion
1/2 cup chopped celery
6 tablespoons chicken soup base
1/4 teaspoon ground white pepper
1/4 cup margarine
1/4 cup all-purpose flour
1 cup cooked white rice
1 cup diced, cooked chicken meat
16 slices lemon
8 egg yolks

STEPS

1. In a large pot, combine the chicken broth, lemon juice, carrots, onions, celery, soup base, and white pepper. Bring to a boil on high, then simmer for 20 minutes.
2. Blend the butter and the flour together. Then gradually add it to the soup mixture. Simmer for 10 minutes more, stirring frequently.
3. Meanwhile, beat the egg yolks until light in color. Gradually add some of the hot soup to the egg yolks, stirring constantly. Return the egg mixture to the soup pot and heat through. Add the rice and chicken. Ladle hot soup into bowls and garnish with lemon slices.

NUTRITION FACTS

Per Serving:

124 calories
protein 7.8g
carbohydrates 9.1g
fat 6.6g
cholesterol 110.3mg
sodium 1236.8mg

Zucchini Pasta

INGREDIENTS

1 (8 ounce) package uncooked pasta shells
1 teaspoon olive oil
1/2 onion, chopped
3 cloves garlic, sliced
1 zucchini, chopped
1/2 teaspoon dried oregano
salt and freshly ground black pepper to taste
1/4 teaspoon crushed red pepper flakes
3/4 cup chicken broth
1/2 cup chopped cooked chicken
1 ounce diced roasted red peppers
2 tablespoons light cream cheese
1/4 cup chopped fresh basil leaves
1/4 cup grated Parmesan cheese

STEPS

1. Bring a large pot of lightly salted water to a boil. Place pasta shells in the pot, cook for 8 to 10 minutes, until al dente, and drain.
2. Heat the olive oil in a skillet over medium heat, and cook the onion and garlic until tender. Mix in the zucchini, and season with oregano, salt and pepper, and red pepper. Cook 10 minutes, until tender.
3. Stir the chicken broth into the skillet, and cook 5 minutes, until heated through. Mix in the chicken, roasted red peppers, and cream cheese, and continue cooking 5 minutes. Serve over the cooked pasta, and top with fresh basil and Parmesan cheese.

NUTRITION FACTS

Per Serving:

321 calories
protein 16.7g
carbohydrates 48.2g
fat 6.6g
cholesterol 21.3mg
sodium 739.4mg

Greek Chicken Salad

SALAD

PREPARATION
15 MIN

SERVES FOR
4 PEOPLE

INGREDIENTS

2 cups cubed, cooked chicken meat
1/2 cup sliced carrots
1/2 cup sliced cucumber
1/4 cup sliced black olives
1/4 cup crumbled feta cheese
1/4 cup Italian-style salad dressing

STEPS

1. In a large bowl combine the chicken, carrots, cucumber, olives and cheese. Gently mix together. Add the salad dressing and mix well.
2. Cover and refrigerate. Let flavors marinate for at least 1 hour. Serve on a bed of lettuce if desired.

NUTRITION FACTS

Per Serving:

193 calories
protein 20.7g
carbohydrates 4.3g
fat 10g
cholesterol 60.8mg
sodium 471.6mg

Spanish Moroccan Fish

PREPARATION
30 MIN

SERVES FOR
12 PEOPLE

INGREDIENTS

1 tablespoon vegetable oil
1 onion, chopped
1 clove garlic, finely chopped
1 (15 ounce) can garbanzo beans, drained and rinsed
2 red bell peppers, seeded and sliced into strips
1 large carrot, thinly sliced
3 tomatoes, chopped
4 olives, chopped
1/4 cup chopped fresh parsley
1/4 cup ground cumin
3 tablespoons paprika
2 tablespoons chicken bouillon granules
1 teaspoon cayenne pepper
salt to taste
5 pounds tilapia fillets

NUTRITION FACTS

Per Serving:

268 calories
protein 41.7g
carbohydrates 12.6g
fat 5.1g
cholesterol 69.6mg
sodium 381.1mg

STEPS

1. Heat vegetable oil in a skillet over medium heat. Stir in onion and garlic; cook and stir until the onion has softened and turned translucent, about 5 minutes. Add garbanzo beans, bell peppers, carrots, tomatoes, and olives; continue to cook until the peppers are slightly tender, about 5 minutes more.

2. Sprinkle parsley, cumin, paprika, chicken bouillon, and cayenne over the vegetables. Season with salt. Stir to incorporate. Place tilapia on top of the vegetables and add enough water to cover the vegetables. Reduce heat to low, cover, and cook until fish flakes easily with a fork and juices run clear, about 40 minutes.

Mediterranean Power Lentil Salad

PREPARATION
10 MIN

SERVES FOR
6 PEOPLE

INGREDIENTS

1 cup dry green lentils or black lentils
Seeds of 1 pomegranate
Water
Kosher salt
1 small red onion chopped
3/4 english cucumber small diced or chopped
(about 2 1/2 cups)
2 to 3 cups baby spinach or other leafy green
of choice
1 cup chopped fresh parsley
Crumbled feta cheese for garnish
Lime Dressing
1/4 cup fresh lime juice
1/3 cup extra virgin olive oil
2 tsp honey
1 tsp ground cumin
1/2 tsp ground allspice
Salt and pepper

NUTRITION FACTS

Per Serving:

431 calories
protein 15.3g
carbohydrates 11.7g
fat 36.1g
cholesterol 138.4mg
sodium 857.4mg

STEPS

1. Bring a large pot of lightly salted water to a boil. Cook gnocchi in the boiling water until they float to the top, 2 to 4 minutes. Drain.
2. Place a steamer insert into a saucepan and fill with water to just below the bottom of the steamer. Bring water to a boil. Add broccoli, cover, and steam until tender, 4 to 5 minutes. Drain and keep warm.
3. Melt 1 teaspoon butter in a large skillet over medium heat. Add 1 tablespoon onion and 1 teaspoon garlic; cook and stir until fragrant, about 2 minutes. Add sausage; cook and stir until browned, about 5 minutes. Stir in broccoli.
4. Melt 1/2 cup butter in another skillet. Add remaining 1 tablespoon onion, 2 teaspoons garlic, and flour; cook and stir until lightly browned, 2 to 3 minutes. Stir in gnocchi.
5. Combine sausage mixture and gnocchi mixture; season with salt and pepper.

Chicken Breast Cutlets with Artichokes and Capers

PREPARATION
20 MIN

SERVES FOR
6 PEOPLE

INGREDIENTS

1 cup whole wheat or white flour
1/2 teaspoon salt
1/8 teaspoon white pepper, or to taste
1/8 teaspoon black pepper, or to taste
2 pounds chicken breast tenderloins or strips
2 tablespoons canola oil
2 tablespoons extra-virgin olive oil
2 cups chicken broth
2 tablespoons fresh lemon juice
1 (12 ounce) jar quartered marinated artichoke hearts, with liquid
1/4 cup capers
2 tablespoons butter
1/4 cup chopped flat-leaf parsley

NUTRITION FACTS

Per Serving:

408 calories
protein 40.1g
carbohydrates 22g
fat 18.6g
cholesterol 97.9mg
sodium 719.3mg

STEPS

1. Combine flour, salt, and white and black peppers. Dredge chicken in seasoned flour and shake off excess.
2. Heat canola oil and olive oil in a large skillet over medium-high heat. Add chicken breasts and cook until golden brown on both sides, and no longer pink on the inside; set aside.
3. Pour in chicken broth and lemon juice. Bring to a simmer, scraping the bottom of the pan to dissolve the caramelized bits. Add artichoke hearts and capers, return to a simmer, and cook until reduced by half.
4. Whisk butter into sauce until melted. Place cooked chicken back into pan, and simmer in the sauce for a few minutes to reheat. Serve on a platter sprinkled with chopped fresh parsley.

Chakchouka (Shakshouka)

INGREDIENTS

3 tablespoons olive oil
11/3 cups chopped onion
1 cup thinly sliced bell peppers, any color
2 cloves garlic, minced, or to taste
2 1/2 cups chopped tomatoes
1 teaspoon ground cumin
1 teaspoon paprika
1 teaspoon salt
1 hot chile pepper, seeded and finely chopped,
or to taste
4 eggs

NUTRITION FACTS

Per Serving:

209 calories
protein 7.8g
carbohydrates 12.9g
fat 15g
cholesterol 163.7mg
sodium 653.7mg

STEPS

1. Heat the olive oil in a skillet over medium heat. Stir in the onion, bell peppers, and garlic; cook and stir until the vegetables have softened and the onion has turned translucent, about 5 minutes.
2. Combine the tomatoes, cumin, paprika, salt, and chile pepper into a bowl and mix briefly. Pour the tomato mixture into the skillet, and stir to combine.
3. Simmer, uncovered, until the tomato juices have cooked off, about 10 minutes. Make four indentations in the tomato mixture for the eggs. Crack the eggs into the indentations. Cover the skillet and let the eggs cook until they're firm but not dry, about 5 minutes.

Mediterranean Cauliflower Pizza

INGREDIENTS

1 pound beef stew meat
salt and ground black pepper to taste
1/2 cup chopped Spanish onion
2 cloves garlic, minced
2 cups chopped red potatoes
1 (14.5 ounce) can diced tomatoes
1 (12 ounce) jar sofrito
1/2 cup pitted and halved green olives

NUTRITION FACTS

Per Serving:

200 calories
protein 10.8g
carbohydrates 10.2g
fat 13.9g
cholesterol 64.9mg
sodium 483.6mg

STEPS

1. Preheat oven to 450 degrees F. Line a pizza pan or rimless baking sheet with parchment paper.
2. Place cauliflower in a food processor and pulse until reduced to rice-size crumbles. Transfer to a large nonstick skillet and add 1 tablespoon oil and salt. Heat over medium-high, stirring frequently, until the cauliflower begins to soften slightly (but don't let it brown), 8 to 10 minutes. Transfer to a large bowl to cool for at least 10 minutes.
3. Remove the skin and white pith from the lemon and discard. Working over a small bowl, cut the segments from the membranes, letting the segments drop into the bowl (remove seeds). Drain the juice from the segments (save for another use). Add tomatoes and olives to the lemon segments; toss to combine.
4. Add egg, cheese and oregano to the cooled cauliflower; stir to combine. Spread the mixture onto the prepared baking sheet, shaping into an even 10-inch round. Drizzle the remaining 1 teaspoon oil over the top.
5. Bake the pizza until the top begins to brown, 10 to 14 minutes. Scatter the lemon- olive mixture over the top, season with pepper, and continue to bake until nicely browned all over, 8 to 14 minutes more. Scatter basil over the top.

Skillet Gnocchi with Chard & White Beans

PREPARATION
30 MIN

SERVES FOR
6 PEOPLE

INGREDIENTS

1 tablespoon extra-virgin olive oil
1 (16 ounce) package shelf-stable gnocchi
1 teaspoon extra-virgin olive oil
1 medium yellow onion, thinly sliced
4 cloves garlic, minced
1/2 cup water
6 cups chopped chard leaves or spinach
1 (15 ounce) can diced tomatoes with Italian seasonings
1 (15 ounce) can white beans, rinsed
1/4 teaspoon freshly ground pepper
1/2 cup shredded part-skim mozzarella cheese
1/4 cup finely shredded Parmesan cheese

STEPS

1. Heat 1 tablespoon oil in a large nonstick skillet over medium heat. Add gnocchi and cook, stirring often, until plumped and starting to brown, 5 to 7 minutes. Transfer to a bowl.

2. Add the remaining 1 teaspoon oil and onion to the pan and cook, stirring, over medium heat, for 2 minutes. Stir in garlic and water. Cover and cook until the onion is soft, 4 to 6 minutes. Add chard (or spinach) and cook, stirring, until starting to wilt, 1 to 2 minutes. Stir in tomatoes, beans and pepper and bring to a simmer. Stir in the gnocchi and sprinkle with mozzarella and Parmesan. Cover and cook until the cheese is melted and the sauce is bubbling, about 3 minutes.

NUTRITION FACTS

Per Serving:

259 calories
protein 9.7g
carbohydrates 29.5g
fat 11.1g
cholesterol 22.6mg
sodium 505.3mg

Caramelized Onion, Olive & Anchovy Socca

PREPARATION
1 HR

SERVES FOR
4 PEOPLE

INGREDIENTS

1 cup chickpea flour
1/2 teaspoon salt
1/4 teaspoon ground black pepper
1 cup water
3 tablespoons extra-virgin olive oil, divided
1 medium onion, thinly sliced
6 anchovies
8 oil-cured olives, pitted and halved
2 teaspoons chopped fresh thyme

NUTRITION FACTS

Per Serving:

230 calories
protein 6.5g
carbohydrates 26.6g
fat 10.9g
cholesterol 5.1mg
sodium 286.2mg

STEPS

1. Whisk flour, salt and pepper in a large bowl. Add water; whisk until smooth. Let rest while the oven preheats or refrigerate for up to 1 day.
2. Position racks in upper and lower thirds of oven. Place a 12-inch cast-iron skillet on the lower rack. Preheat to 450 degrees F for 30 minutes.
3. Meanwhile, heat 1 tablespoon oil in a medium skillet over medium-high heat. Add onion and cook, stirring occasionally, until starting to brown, about 5 minutes. Reduce heat to medium and cook, stirring occasionally, until golden, about 6 minutes more, adding a tablespoon or two of water, if needed, to prevent burning.
4. When the oven is preheated, carefully remove the hot pan and swirl in 1 tablespoon oil. Whisk the batter, pour it into the pan and swirl to coat. Top with the onion, anchovies and olives.
5. Bake until the bottom is browned and the edges are crispy, 16 to 20 minutes. Remove from the oven and, using a pastry brush, dab the socca with the remaining 1 tablespoon oil (brushing can dislodge the toppings).
6. Turn the broiler to high. Broil the socca on the upper rack until browned in spots, 1 to 3 minutes.

Fasolakia
(Greek Green Beans)

PREPARATION
15 MIN

SERVES FOR
4 PEOPLE

INGREDIENTS

1/4 cup olive oil
1 small onion, grated
1 1/2 pounds fresh green beans, trimmed
4 tomatoes, pureed
2 yellow potatoes, peeled and cut into wedges
1/2 teaspoon salt, or to taste
ground black pepper to taste
1 pinch white sugar
water to cover

STEPS

1. Heat olive oil in a large saucepan over medium heat and stir in onion. Cook until onion has softened, about 5 minutes. Add green beans and stir to coat in the oil. Cook, stirring occasionally, 2 to 3 minutes. Add pureed tomato, potatoes, salt, pepper, and sugar. Stir well, then add water until beans are barely covered.

2. Bring to a simmer, partially cover with a lid, and cook gently over medium-low heat until green beans and potatoes are soft, 25 to 30 minutes. Uncover towards the end of cooking to reduce sauce if it is too watery.

NUTRITION FACTS

Per Serving:

289 calories
protein 6.8g
carbohydrates 38.6g
fat 14.1g
sodium 316.7mg

Black Bass with Sautéed Vegetables & Cioppino Jus

INGREDIENTS

1 pound unpeeled, head-on raw shrimp
4 tablespoons canola oil, divided
1/3 cup chopped onion
3 cloves garlic, smashed
1 cup chopped fennel
1/2 cup chopped carrot
1/2 cup chopped celery
1/3 cup tomato paste
1/2 cup Pernod or other pastis, plus 2 table-spoons, divided
8 cups water
1 bay leaf
2 sprigs fresh thyme
1 teaspoon crushed red pepper
1 teaspoon whole peppercorns
3/4 teaspoon kosher salt, divided
1 medium yellow squash, diced
1 medium medium zucchini, diced
15 cherry tomatoes, halved
2 tablespoons butter, divided
1 teaspoon ground pepper
4 (5 ounce) skin-on black bass or cod fillets
Chopped fennel fronds, fresh tarragon, lemon zest & fennel pollen for garnish

NUTRITION FACTS

Per Serving:

383 calories
protein 34.7g
carbohydrates 14.7g
fat 18.1g
cholesterol 116.6mg
sodium 614mg

STEPS

1. Preheat oven to 350 degrees F. Coat a 9-by-13-inch baking pan with cooking spray.
2. Twist heads off shrimp and place the heads in the prepared pan. Pull off and discard legs. Peel and devein the shrimp; set the shrimp aside in the refrigerator and add the shells to the pan. Roast the heads and shells until pink and crispy, about 15 minutes.
3. Meanwhile, heat 1 1/2 tablespoons oil in a large pot over medium-low heat. Add onion and garlic and cook, stirring occasionally, until translucent, about 5 minutes. Add fennel, carrot and celery and cook, stirring occasionally, until softened, about 8 minutes. Add tomato paste and cook, stirring, until fragrant, about 1 minute. Add 1/2 cup Pernod (or other pastis) and cook, stirring, until the liquid has evaporated, about 1 minute.
4. Add water, bay leaf, thyme, crushed red pepper, pepper-corns, the roasted heads and shells and the reserved shrimp. Bring to a boil over high heat. Reduce heat to maintain a lively simmer and cook, stirring occa-sionally, until reduced to 6 cups, 1 to 1 1/2 hours.

5. Discard the bay leaf. Transfer the mixture to a blender in batches and blend until smooth (be careful when blending hot liquids). Pour through a fine-mesh sieve into a large saucepan, pressing on the solids to get as much liquid as possible. (You should have about 4 cups of cioppino jus.) Season with 1/2 teaspoon salt. Cover to keep warm.

6. Heat 1 1/2 tablespoons oil in a large skillet over medium heat. Add squash and zucchini and cook, stirring occasionally, until starting to brown, 10 to 12 minutes. Stir in tomatoes, then the remaining 2 tablespoons Pernod (or other pastis), scraping up any browned bits. Stir in 1 tablespoon butter and pepper. Cover to keep warm.

7. Pat fish dry with paper towels and sprinkle with the remaining 1/4 teaspoon salt. Heat the remaining 1 tablespoon oil in a large nonstick skillet over medium-high heat. Add the fish, skin-side down. Cook, pressing gently with a spatula, until the skin is crispy, about 5 minutes. Turn the fish and add the remaining 1 tablespoon butter. Cook, basting with the butter, until the fish is just cooked through, 3 to 5 minutes more.

8. Divide the vegetables among 4 shallow bowls and top each with a piece of fish. Pour 1/4 cup cioppino jus around the vegetables. Garnish with fennel fronds, tarragon, lemon zest and fennel pollen, if desired.

Lemon Chicken Orzo Soup

PREPARATION
20 MIN

SERVES FOR
12 PEOPLE

INGREDIENTS

8 ounces orzo pasta
1 teaspoon olive oil
3 carrots, chopped, or more to taste
3 ribs celery, chopped
1 onion, chopped
2 cloves garlic, minced
1/2 teaspoon dried thyme
1/2 teaspoon dried oregano
salt and ground black pepper to taste
1 bay leaf
3 (32 ounce) cartons fat-free, low-sodium chicken broth
1/2 cup fresh lemon juice
1 lemon, zested
8 ounces cooked chicken breast, chopped
1 (8 ounce) package baby spinach leaves
1 lemon, sliced for garnish
1/4 cup grated Parmesan cheese

NUTRITION FACTS

Per Serving:
Calories: 141.2kcal
Carbohydrates: 11.8g
Protein: 9.2g
Saturated Fat: 0.3g
Fiber: 2.3g

STEPS

1. Bring a large pot of lightly salted water to a boil. Cook orzo in the boiling water until partially cooked through but not yet soft, about 5 minutes; drain and rinse with cold water until cooled completely.
2. Heat olive oil in a large pot over medium heat. Cook and stir carrots, celery, and onion in hot oil until the vegetables begin to soften and the onion becomes translucent, 5 to 7 minutes. Add garlic; cook and stir until fragrant, about 1 minute more. Season mixture with thyme, oregano, salt, black pepper, and bay leaf; continue cooking another 30 seconds before pouring chicken broth into the pot.
3. Bring the broth to a boil. Partially cover the pot, reduce heat to medium-low, and simmer until the vegetables are just tender, about 10 minutes.
4. Stir orzo, lemon juice, and lemon zest into the broth; add chicken. Cook until the chicken and orzo are heated through, about 5 minutes. Add baby spinach; cook until the spinach wilts into the broth and the orzo is tender, 2 to 3 minutes. Ladle soup into bowls.

Chicken Tenders with Balsamic-Fig Sauce

PREPARATION
15 MIN

SERVES FOR
4 PEOPLE

INGREDIENTS

1 pound chicken tenders
salt and ground black pepper to taste
1/4 cup all-purpose flour
2 tablespoons olive oil
1 tablespoon butter
Sauce:
1 shallot, minced
1 clove garlic, minced
1/2 cup red wine
1/4 cup balsamic vinegar
4 fresh figs, cut into 1/2-inch pieces
1 teaspoon minced fresh thyme leaves
1 teaspoon Dijon mustard
1 teaspoon honey
1/2 teaspoon salt
1 teaspoon butter

STEPS

1. Season chicken with salt and pepper on both sides and lightly coat with flour, shaking off excess.
2. Heat olive oil and butter in a large nonstick skillet over medium heat. Add chicken to the skillet and cook until tenders are golden brown, no longer pink in the centers, and juices run clear, 5 to 6 minutes, flipping halfway through. Transfer to a plate and cover loosely with aluminum foil to keep warm.
3. Add shallot and garlic to the same skillet and cook until softened, about 2 minutes. Add red wine and balsamic and let simmer until reduced by half, 3 to 5 minutes. Stir in figs, thyme, Dijon mustard, honey, and salt; bring to a boil. Reduce heat to low or medium-low and let simmer until thickened, about 3 minutes. Remove from heat and stir in butter.
4. Spoon sauce over warm chicken tenders, or add chicken back into the skillet to briefly reheat, and serve immediately.

NUTRITION FACTS

Per Serving:

354 calories
protein 27.1g
carbohydrates 23.2g
fat 14.5g
cholesterol 79.5mg
sodium 455.9mg

One-Pot Mediterranean Chicken

PREPARATION
15 MIN

SERVES FOR
6 PEOPLE

INGREDIENTS

1 stick butter
1/2 cup chopped onions
1 tablespoon minced garlic
1 teaspoon Italian seasoning
1/2 teaspoon dried basil
salt to taste
2 (14 ounce) cans artichoke hearts, drained and quartered
1 (28 ounce) can crushed tomatoes
1 (14.5 ounce) can diced tomatoes
1 (6 ounce) can black olives, halved
1 (4.5 ounce) can sliced mushrooms, drained
4 boneless, skinless chicken breasts

STEPS

1. Melt butter in a large skillet over medium-high heat. Add onions, garlic, Italian seasoning, basil, and salt. Saute until it starts to brown, about 5 minutes.
2. Add artichoke hearts, crushed tomatoes, diced tomatoes, olives, and mushrooms; bring to a boil. Add chicken, cover, and reduce heat to medium. Cook, stirring occasionally, until chicken is cooked through and the juices run clear, about 20 to 25 minutes.

NUTRITION FACTS

Per Serving:

361 calories
protein 20.3g
carbohydrates 23.5g
fat 20.6g
cholesterol 79.7mg
sodium 1400.6mg

Easy Skillet Chicken Primavera

PREPARATION
20 MIN

SERVES FOR
6 PEOPLE

INGREDIENTS

1/2 cup all-purpose flour
1 tablespoon dried parsley
1 teaspoon dried basil
1 1/2 pounds skinless, boneless chicken breasts, cut into strips
1/4 cup extra-virgin olive oil
1 tablespoon minced garlic
2 1/4 cups low-sodium chicken stock
1 cup frozen mixed vegetables
1 pint grape tomatoes, halved
1 bunch green onions, diagonally sliced
1 medium zucchini, quartered and sliced
2 tablespoons sun-dried tomato pesto
salt and ground black pepper to taste

cook, turning occasionally, until lightly browned on the outside and no longer pink, about 10 minutes. Add garlic and cook for 1 minute.
3.   Add chicken stock, mixed vegetables, grape tomatoes, green onions, zucchini, and pesto. Cook, stirring occasionally, until heated through, about 10 minutes.

STEPS

1.   Whisk together flour, parsley, and basil in a medium bowl. Add chicken strips and toss until well coated.
2.   Heat olive oil in a large skillet over medium heat. Add chicken and

NUTRITION FACTS

Per Serving:

302 calories
protein 26.3g
carbohydrates 19.4g
fat 13.3g
cholesterol 60.8mg
sodium 544mg

Pollo al Ajillo (Spanish Garlic Chicken)

PREPARATION
20 MIN

SERVES FOR
4 PEOPLE

INGREDIENTS

1 (2 to 3 pound) bone-in chicken, cut into pieces, skin removed
2 tablespoons all-purpose flour, or as needed
5 tablespoons extra-virgin olive oil
salt to taste
6 cloves garlic, chopped
2 bunches fresh basil, chopped
1 cup dry white wine
1 lemon, juiced

STEPS

1. Lightly coat chicken with flour on all sides.
2. Heat oil in a heavy, large skillet over medium-high heat and cook chicken in batches until browned, 5 to 10 minutes per batch. Season with salt and remove chicken pieces from skillet. Add garlic and basil to the same oil in the skillet and cook for 2 minutes.
3. Return chicken pieces to the skillet and add white wine. Cover and simmer over low heat until chicken is cooked through and the juices run clear, about 30 minutes. Add lemon juice just before serving.

NUTRITION FACTS

Per Serving:

542 calories
protein 48.5g
carbohydrates 10.1g
fat 29.1g
cholesterol 142mg
sodium 182.4mg

Simple Shrimp Chowder

PREPARATION
30 MIN

SERVES FOR
5 PEOPLE

INGREDIENTS

1/2 cup each chopped onion, celery, carrot and sweet red pepper
1/4 cup butter, cubed
1/4 cup all-purpose flour
2 cups 2% milk
1/2 pound cooked small shrimp, peeled and deveined
1 can (14-1/2 ounces) diced potatoes, drained
1 cup vegetable broth
1 cup frozen corn, thawed
2 teaspoons seafood seasoning
1 teaspoon minced fresh thyme or 1/2 teaspoon dried thyme
Additional minced fresh thyme

STEPS

1. In a large saucepan, saute the onion, celery, carrot and red pepper in butter for 5 minutes or until tender. Stir in flour until blended; gradually add milk. Bring to a boil; cook and stir for 2 minutes or until thickened.
2. Add the shrimp, potatoes, broth, corn, seafood seasoning and thyme. Reduce heat; cover and simmer for 10 minutes or until heated through. If desired, top with additional minced fresh thyme.

NUTRITION FACTS

Per Serving:

268 calories
protein 16g
carbohydrates 25g
fat 12g
cholesterol 120mg
sodium 901mg

Italian White Bean Chicken

PREPARATION
20 MIN

SERVES FOR
2 PEOPLE

INGREDIENTS

1 clove garlic, sliced
2 skinless, boneless chicken breast halves
2 zucchinis, sliced
1 (15.5 ounce) can white beans, drained
1 roma tomato, chopped
5 fresh basil leaves
ground black pepper to taste

STEPS

1. Prepare a skillet with cooking spray and place over medium heat. Cook the garlic in the skillet until browned. Add the chicken and cook until slightly browned, about 3 minutes per side. Stir the zucchini and white beans into the skillet; cover and cook about 5 minutes. Scatter the tomato over the dish; cover again and cook another 2 minutes. Add the basil leaves and cook 1 minute more. Season with black pepper to serve.

NUTRITION FACTS

Per Serving:

430 calories
protein 44g
carbohydrates 55g
fat 4.7g
cholesterol 69.2mg
sodium 92.6mg

Slow Cooker Mediterranean Chicken and Vegetables

PREPARATION
30 MIN

SERVES FOR
8 PEOPLE

INGREDIENTS

1 teaspoon ground turmeric
1 teaspoon ground ginger
1 teaspoon ground coriander
1 teaspoon salt
1/4 teaspoon ground cumin
1/4 teaspoon cayenne pepper
8 bone-in chicken thighs, skin removed
1 (15 ounce) can chickpeas, drained
1 (14.5 ounce) can diced tomatoes, undrained
12 marinated artichoke hearts, drained
4 large carrots, chopped
4 large garlic cloves, halved
1 (3 inch) piece cinnamon stick
1 tablespoon olive oil, or more as needed
1 large sweet onion, halved and thinly sliced
1/2 pound green beans, trimmed and halved
1 red bell pepper, seeded and cut into 1-inch pieces
1/4 cup coarsely chopped cilantro
3 cups water
2 cups couscous

NUTRITION FACTS

Per Serving:

841 calories
protein 68.1g
carbohydrates 13.8g
fat 55.9g
cholesterol 248.7mg
sodium 2694.3mg

STEPS

1. Combine turmeric, ginger, coriander, salt, cumin, and cayenne pepper in a small cup. Rub mixture over chicken and let sit at least 30 minutes.
2. Combine chickpeas, diced tomatoes, artichoke hearts, carrots, garlic, and cinnamon stick in the bottom of a 6- to 7-quart slow cooker.
3. Heat olive oil in a large nonstick skillet over medium-high heat. Add chicken and brown, about 4 minutes per side. Transfer chicken to the slow cooker, bone-side-up. Add onion to the same skillet. Saute over medium-high heat until onions have taken on a yellow color from turmeric and are starting to brown on the edges, about 5 minutes. Transfer to the slow cooker.
4. Cover the slow cooker and cook on Low for approximately 2 hr.
5. Place green beans and bell pepper over chicken. Cover and cook approximately 3 hr more.
6. Meanwhile, boil 3 cups of water in a saucepan. Add couscous and stir. Cover the pot and turn off the heat. Let sit until water is absorbed and couscous is tender, 5 to 10 minutes.
7. Place hot couscous on each plate and top with chicken and vegetables. Spoon juices from the slow cooker over each serving.

Poached Eggs Caprese

PREPARATION
10 MIN

SERVES FOR
2 PEOPLE

INGREDIENTS

1 tablespoon distilled white vinegar
2 teaspoons salt
4 eggs
2 English muffin, split
4 (1 ounce) slices mozzarella cheese
1 tomato, thickly sliced
4 teaspoons pesto
salt to taste

NUTRITION FACTS

Per Serving:

482 calories
protein 33.3g
carbohydrates 31.7g
fat 24.9g
cholesterol 411.6mg
sodium 3092.7mg

STEPS

1. Fill a large saucepan with 2 to 3 inches of water and bring to a boil over high heat. Reduce the heat to medium-low, pour in the vinegar and 2 teaspoons of salt, and keep the water at a gentle simmer.

2. While waiting for the water to simmer, place a slice of mozzarella cheese and a thick slice of tomato onto each English muffin half, and toast in a toaster oven until the cheese softens and the English muffin has toasted, about 5 minutes.

3. Crack an egg into a small bowl. Holding the bowl just above the surface of the water, gently slip the egg into the simmering water. Repeat with the remaining eggs. Poach the eggs until the whites are firm and the yolks have thickened but are not hard, 2 1/2 to 3 minutes. Remove the eggs from the water with a slotted spoon, and dab on a kitchen towel to remove excess water.

4. To assemble, place a poached egg on top of each English muffin. Spoon a teaspoon of pesto sauce onto each egg and sprinkle with salt to taste.

Eggs and Greens Breakfast Dish

PREPARATION
10 MIN

SERVES FOR
2 PEOPLE

INGREDIENTS

1 tablespoon olive oil
2 cups stemmed and chopped rainbow chard
1 cup fresh spinach
1/2 cup arugula
2 cloves garlic, minced
4 eggs, beaten
1/2 cup shredded Cheddar cheese
salt and ground black pepper to taste

STEPS

1. Heat oil in a skillet over medium-high heat. Saute chard, spinach, and arugula until tender, about 3 minutes. Add garlic; cook and stir until fragrant, about 2 minutes.
2. Mix eggs and cheese together in a bowl; pour into the chard mixture. Cover and cook until set, 5 to 7 minutes. Season with salt and pepper.

NUTRITION FACTS

Per Serving:

333 calories
protein 21g
carbohydrates 4.2g
fat 26.2g
cholesterol 401.7mg
sodium 483.5mg

Breakfast Pita Pizza

PREPARATION
25 MIN

SERVES FOR
2 PEOPLE

INGREDIENTS

4 slices bacon
1/4 onion, chopped
2 tablespoons extra-virgin olive oil
4 eggs, beaten
2 tablespoons pesto
2 pita bread rounds
1/2 tomato, chopped
1/4 cup chopped fresh mushrooms
1/2 cup chopped spinach
1/2 cup shredded Cheddar cheese
1 avocado - peeled, pitted, and sliced

NUTRITION FACTS

Per Serving:

873 calories
protein 36.8g
carbohydrates 43.5g
fat 62.9g
cholesterol 426.5mg
sodium 1134.6mg

STEPS

1. Preheat oven to 350 degrees F (175 degrees C). Line a baking sheet with parchment paper.
2. Place bacon in a large skillet and cook over medium-high heat, turning occasionally, until evenly browned, about 10 minutes. Drain on paper towels. Cook and stir onion in the same skillet until soft and translucent, about 5 minutes. Remove and set aside. Heat olive oil in the skillet. Pour in eggs and cook, stirring occasionally, until set, 3 to 5 minutes.
3. Place pita bread on lined baking sheet. Spread pesto over pita; top with bacon, scrambled eggs, tomato, mushrooms, and spinach. Sprinkle Cheddar cheese over toppings.
4. Bake in the preheated oven until cheese has melted, about 10 minutes. Serve garnished with avocado slices.

Caprese on Toast

PREPARATION
15 MIN

SERVES FOR
14 PEOPLE

INGREDIENTS

14 slices sourdough bread
2 cloves garlic, peeled
1 pound fresh mozzarella cheese, sliced 1/4-inch thick
1/3 cup fresh basil leaves
3 large tomatoes, sliced 1/4-inch thick
3 tablespoons extra-virgin olive oil
salt and ground black pepper to taste

STEPS

1. Toast bread slices and rub one side of each slice with garlic. Place a slice of mozzarella cheese, 1 to 2 basil leaves, and a slice of tomato on each piece of toast. Drizzle with olive oil and season with salt and black pepper.

NUTRITION FACTS

Per Serving:

204 calories
protein 10.5g
carbohydrates 16.5g
fat 10.7g
cholesterol 25.6mg
sodium 367.9mg

Mediterranean Breakfast Quinoa

PREPARATION
10 MIN

SERVES FOR
4 PEOPLE

INGREDIENTS

1/4 cup chopped raw almonds
1 teaspoon ground cinnamon
1 cup quinoa
2 cups milk
1 teaspoon sea salt
1 teaspoon vanilla extract
2 tablespoons honey
2 dried pitted dates, finely chopped
5 dried apricots, finely chopped

STEPS

1. Toast the almonds in a skillet over medium heat until just golden, 3 to 5 minutes; set aside.
2. Heat the cinnamon and quinoa together in a saucepan over medium heat until warmed through. Add the milk and sea salt to the saucepan and stir; bring the mixture to a boil, reduce heat to low, place a cover on the saucepan, and allow to cook at a simmer for 15 minutes. Stir the vanilla, honey, dates, apricots, and about half the almonds into the quinoa mixture. Top with the remaining almonds to serve.

NUTRITION FACTS

Per Serving:

327 calories
protein 11.5g
carbohydrates 53.9g
fat 7.9g
cholesterol 9.8mg
sodium 500.9mg

Eggs Florentine

PREPARATION
10 MIN

SERVES FOR
3 PEOPLE

INGREDIENTS

2 tablespoons butter
1/2 cup mushrooms, sliced
2 cloves garlic, minced
1/2 (10 ounce) package fresh spinach
6 large eggs, slightly beaten
salt and ground black pepper to taste
3 tablespoons cream cheese, cut into small pieces

STEPS

1. Melt butter in a large skillet over medium heat; cook and stir mushrooms and garlic until garlic is fragrant, about 1 minute. Add spinach to mushroom mixture and cook until spinach is wilted, 2 to 3 minutes.
2. Stir eggs into mushroom-spinach mixture; season with salt and pepper. Cook, without stirring, until eggs start to firm; flip. Sprinkle cream cheese over egg mixture and cook until cream cheese starts to soften, about 5 minutes.

NUTRITION FACTS

Per Serving:

279 calories
protein 15.7g
carbohydrates 4.1g
fat 22.9g
cholesterol 408.3mg
sodium 276mg

Speedy Salmon Patties

PREPARATION
25 MIN

SERVES FOR
3 PEOPLE

INGREDIENTS

1/3 cup finely chopped onion
1 large egg, beaten
5 saltines, crushed
1/2 teaspoon Worcestershire sauce
1/4 teaspoon salt
1/8 teaspoon pepper
1 can (14-3/4 ounces) salmon, drained, bones and skin removed
2 teaspoons butter

STEPS

1. In a large bowl, combine the first 6 ingredients. Crumble salmon over mixture and mix well. Shape into 6 patties.
2. In a large skillet over medium heat, fry patties in butter for 3-4 minutes on each side or until set and golden brown.

NUTRITION FACTS

Per Serving:

288 calories
protein 31g
carbohydrates 5g
fat 15g
cholesterol 139mg
sodium 1063mg

Quinoa Breakfast Cereal

PREPARATION
5 MIN

SERVES FOR
4 PEOPLE

INGREDIENTS

2 cups water
1 cup quinoa, rinsed
1/2 cup chopped dried apricots
1/2 cup slivered almonds
1/3 cup flax seeds
1 teaspoon ground cinnamon
1/2 teaspoon ground nutmeg

STEPS

1. Combine water and quinoa in a saucepan over medium heat; bring to a boil. Reduce heat and simmer until most of the water has been absorbed, 8 to 12 minutes. Stir in apricots, almonds, flax seeds, cinnamon, and nutmeg; cook until quinoa is tender, 2 to 3 minutes more.

NUTRITION FACTS

Per Serving:

350 calories
protein 11.8g
carbohydrates 44.5g
fat 15.1g
sodium 12.8mg

Healthy Breakfast Sandwich

PREPARATION
5 MIN

SERVES FOR
2 PEOPLE

INGREDIENTS

3/4 cup liquid egg whites
2 whole-wheat English muffins, split
1/2 cup baby spinach leaves
2 slices fresh tomato

STEPS

1. Cook egg whites in a nonstick skillet over medium heat until opaque, about 4 minutes.
2. Toast English muffins. Divide cooked egg whites between 2 muffin bottoms. Top with spinach, 1 tomato slice, and muffin tops.

NUTRITION FACTS

Per Serving:

186 calories
protein 16.3g
carbohydrates 28.8g
fat 1.5g
sodium 474mg

Spinach Feta Egg Wrap

PREPARATION
10 MIN

SERVES FOR
1 PEOPLE

INGREDIENTS

1 large whole-wheat tortilla
1 1/2 teaspoons coconut oil
1 cup chopped baby spinach leaves
1 oil-packed sun-dried tomato, chopped
2 eggs, beaten
1/3 cup feta cheese
1 tomato, diced

STEPS

1. Warm tortilla in a large skillet over medium heat.
2. Melt coconut oil in a separate skillet over medium-high heat. Saute spinach and tomato in hot oil until spinach wilts, about 1 minute. Add eggs and scramble until almost set, about 2 minutes. Sprinkle feta cheese over eggs and continue cooking until cheese melts, about 1 minute more.
3. Transfer scrambled egg mixture to warm tortilla in the large skillet; top with diced tomato. Roll tortilla and leave in skillet long enough for wrap to hold its shape, about 30 seconds.

NUTRITION FACTS

Per Serving:

704 calories
protein 36.6g
carbohydrates 78g
fat 36.8g
cholesterol 446.8mg
sodium 1721.5mg

Zucchini with Egg

PREPARATION
5 MIN

SERVES FOR
2 PEOPLE

INGREDIENTS

1 1/2 tablespoons olive oil
2 large zucchini, cut into large chunks
salt and ground black pepper to taste
2 large eggs
1 teaspoon water, or as desired

STEPS

1. Heat oil in a skillet over medium-high heat; saute zucchini until tender, about 10 minutes. Season zucchini with salt and black pepper.
2. Beat eggs with a fork in a bowl; add water and beat until evenly combined. Pour eggs over zucchini; cook and stir until eggs are scrambled and no longer runny, about 5 minutes. Season zucchini and eggs with salt and black pepper.

NUTRITION FACTS

Per Serving:

213 calories
protein 10.2g
carbohydrates 11.2g
fat 15.7g
cholesterol 186mg
sodium 180mg

Paleo Baked Eggs in Avocado

PREPARATION
5 MIN

SERVES FOR
2 PEOPLE

INGREDIENTS

2 small eggs
1 avocado, halved and pitted
2 slices cooked bacon, crumbled
2 teaspoons chopped fresh chives, or to taste
1 pinch dried parsley, or to taste
1 pinch sea salt and ground black pepper to taste

STEPS

1. Preheat oven to 425 degrees F (220 degrees C).
2. Crack the eggs into a bowl, being careful to keep the yolks intact.
3. Arrange avocado halves in a baking dish, resting them along the edge so avocado won't tip over. Gently spoon 1 egg yolk into the avocado hole. Continue spooning egg white into the hole until full. Repeat with remaining egg yolk, egg white, and avocado. Season each filled avocado with chives, parsley, sea salt, and pepper.
4. Gently place baking dish in the preheated oven and bake until eggs are cooked, about 15 minutes. Sprinkle bacon over avocado.

NUTRITION FACTS

Per Serving:

280 calories
protein 11.3g
carbohydrates 9.3g
fat 23.5g
cholesterol 150.8mg
sodium 498.3mg

Scrumptious Breakfast Salad

PREPARATION
35 MIN

SERVES FOR
4 PEOPLE

INGREDIENTS

5 eggs
1 head romaine lettuce, chopped
2 avocados, sliced
2 large tomatoes, sliced
1 pint fresh strawberries, sliced
4 clementines, peeled and segmented
1 Spanish onion, sliced into rounds
1 ripe mango, peeled and sliced
1 Pink Lady apple, diced
1 nectarine, sliced
1 cucumber, diced
1/4 cup vinaigrette salad dressing, or to taste

STEPS

1. Place eggs in a saucepan and cover with water. Bring to a boil, remove from heat, and let eggs stand in hot water for 15 minutes.
2. Layer lettuce, avocados, tomatoes, strawberries, clementines, onion, mango, apple, nectarine, and cucumber in a large bowl or on individual serving plates. Drizzle vinaigrette on top.
3. Remove eggs from hot water; cool under cold running water. Peel and chop. Scatter eggs over the salad.

NUTRITION FACTS

Per Serving:

448 calories
protein 13.4g
carbohydrates 53.7g
fat 24.2g
cholesterol 204.6mg
sodium 234.1mg

Socca (Farinata)

PREPARATION
10 MIN

SERVES FOR
4 PEOPLE

INGREDIENTS

1 cup chickpea flour
1 cup water
1 tablespoon olive oil
1/2 teaspoon ground cumin
salt and ground black pepper to taste
1 tablespoon vegetable oil for frying

STEPS

1. Combine chickpea flour, water, and olive oil in a bowl. Season with cumin, salt, and pepper to taste. Stir everything together until smooth. Set aside and let rest at room temperature for 2 hours.
2. Preheat the oven to 450 degrees F (230 degrees C). Place a cast iron skillet in the oven until hot, 5 to 7 minutes.
3. Carefully remove skillet from oven, grease with oil and pour half of the the batter into the skillet, tilting so batter is evenly distributed.
4. Bake in the preheated oven until socca is set, about 7 minutes. Turn on broiler and brown for 1 minute. Remove from oven and slide onto a plate. Repeat with remaining batter.

NUTRITION FACTS

Per Serving:

146 calories
protein 4.7g
carbohydrates 13.8g
fat 8.4g
sodium 41mg

Blueberry Lemon Breakfast Quinoa

PREPARATION
5 MIN

SERVES FOR
2 PEOPLE

INGREDIENTS

1 cup quinoa
2 cups nonfat milk
1 pinch salt
3 tablespoons maple syrup
1/2 lemon, zested
1 cup blueberries
2 teaspoons flax seed

STEPS

1. Rinse quinoa in a fine strainer with cold water to remove bitterness until water runs clear and is no longer frothy.
2. Heat milk in a saucepan over medium heat until warm, 2 to 3 minutes. Stir quinoa and salt into the milk; simmer over medium-low heat until much of the liquid has been absorbed, about 20 minutes. Remove saucepan from heat. Stir maple syrup and lemon zest into the quinoa mixture. Gently fold blueberries into the mixture.
3. Divide quinoa mixture between 2 bowls; top each with 1 teaspoon flax seed to serve.

NUTRITION FACTS

Per Serving:

538 calories
protein 21.5g
carbohydrates 98.7g
fat 7.3g
cholesterol 4.9mg
sodium 111.9mg

Briam (Greek Baked Zucchini and Potatoes)

PREPARATION
30 MIN

SERVES FOR
4 PEOPLE

INGREDIENTS

2 pounds potatoes, peeled and thinly sliced
4 large zucchini, thinly sliced
4 small red onions, thinly sliced
6 ripe tomatoes, pureed
1/2 cup olive oil
2 tablespoons chopped fresh parsley
sea salt and freshly ground black pepper to taste

STEPS

1. Preheat oven to 400 degrees F (200 degrees C).
2. Spread potatoes, zucchini, and red onions in a 9x13-inch baking dish, or preferably a larger one. Use 2 baking dishes if necessary. Cover with pureed tomatoes, olive oil, parsley. Season with salt and freshly ground pepper. Toss all ingredients together so that the vegetables are evenly coated.
3. Bake in the preheated oven, stirring after 1 hour, until vegetables are tender and moisture has evaporated, about 90 minutes. Cool slightly before serving, or serve at room temperature.

NUTRITION FACTS

Per Serving:

534 calories
protein 11.3g
carbohydrates 65.8g
fat 28.3g
sodium 141.4mg

Slow Cooker Mediterranean Chicken and Vegetables

PREPARATION
30 MIN

SERVES FOR
8 PEOPLE

INGREDIENTS

1 teaspoon ground turmeric
1 teaspoon ground ginger
1 teaspoon ground coriander
1 teaspoon salt
1/4 teaspoon ground cumin
1/4 teaspoon cayenne pepper
8 bone-in chicken thighs, skin removed
1 (15 ounce) can chickpeas, drained
1 (14.5 ounce) can diced tomatoes, undrained
12 marinated artichoke hearts, drained
4 large carrots, chopped
4 large garlic cloves, halved
1 (3 inch) piece cinnamon stick
1 tablespoon olive oil, or more as needed
1 large sweet onion, halved and thinly sliced
1/2 pound green beans, trimmed and halved
1 red bell pepper, seeded and cut into 1-inch pieces
1/4 cup coarsely chopped cilantro
3 cups water
2 cups couscous

NUTRITION FACTS

Per Serving:

465 calories
protein 29.8g
carbohydrates 57.3g
fat 13g
cholesterol 70.3mg
sodium 733.9mg

STEPS

1. Combine turmeric, ginger, coriander, salt, cumin, and cayenne pepper in a small cup. Rub mixture over chicken and let sit at least 30 minutes.
2. Combine chickpeas, diced tomatoes, artichoke hearts, carrots, garlic, and cinnamon stick in the bottom of a 6- to 7-quart slow cooker.
3. Heat olive oil in a large nonstick skillet over medium-high heat. Add chicken and brown, about 4 minutes per side. Transfer chicken to the slow cooker, bone-side-up. Add onion to the same skillet. Saute over medium-high heat until onions have taken on a yellow color from turmeric and are starting to brown on the edges, about 5 minutes. Transfer to the slow cooker.
4. Cover the slow cooker and cook on low for approximately 2 hr.
5. Place green beans and bell pepper over chicken. Cover and cook approximately 3 hr more.
6. Meanwhile, boil 3 cups of water in a saucepan. Add couscous and stir. Cover the pot and turn off the heat. Let sit until water is absorbed and couscous is tender, 5 to 10 minutes.
7. Place hot couscous on each plate and top with chicken and vegetables. Spoon juices from the slow cooker over each serving.

Tuscan Fish Stew

PREPARATION
25 MIN

SERVES FOR
2 PEOPLE

INGREDIENTS

3 cups cherry tomatoes, halved
1 cup clam juice
4 tablespoons olive oil, divided
1/4 cup sliced green onions
4 cloves garlic, sliced
1 anchovy fillet
2 pinches red pepper flakes
12 ounces halibut, cut into 2-inch pieces
1 pound shrimp, peeled and deveined
salt to taste
1 tablespoon chopped fresh parsley
1/2 tablespoon chopped fresh basil
1/2 tablespoon chopped fresh oregano
1 pinch minced fresh rosemary

NUTRITION FACTS

Per Serving:

672 calories
protein 76.3g
carbohydrates 14.3g
fat 34.1g
cholesterol 405mg
sodium 922.4mg

STEPS

1. Puree cherry tomatoes and clam juice in a blender until smooth. Press mixture through a fine-mesh strainer into a bowl.

2. Combine 3 tablespoons olive oil, green onions, garlic, anchovy, and 1 pinch red pepper flakes in a cold plan. Place over medium heat. Cook and stir until garlic and onions just start to soften, about 3 minutes. Stir in the tomato mixture. Bring to a simmer over medium-high heat. Reduce heat to medium and simmer stew until color deepens, about 10 minutes.

3. Add halibut and shrimp to the stew. Season with salt. Increase heat to high. Cover pan and cook until fish flakes easily with a fork, about 5 minutes. Stir in parsley, basil, oregano, and rosemary. Pour stew into a warm bowl. Drizzle in remaining olive oil and sprinkle 1 pinch red pepper flakes on top. Serve with crusty bread.

Mediterranean Chicken and Pepper Casserole

PREPARATION
15 MIN

SERVES FOR
2 PEOPLE

INGREDIENTS

3 cups uncooked mafalda pasta
1 tablespoon olive oil
1 skinless, boneless chicken breast, cut into strips
1 small yellow onion, diced
1 small yellow bell pepper, diced
1 small red bell pepper, diced
8 cherry tomatoes
1/4 cup Italian green olives
1 tablespoon fresh thyme leaves
1 teaspoon grated lemon zest
1/2 teaspoon red pepper flakes
1/4 cup grated Pecorino Romano cheese
1/4 cup grated Grana Padano cheese

NUTRITION FACTS

Per Serving:

479 calories
protein 28.3g
carbohydrates 53.4g
fat 17.8g
cholesterol 53.4mg
sodium 697.8mg

STEPS

1. Preheat the oven to 350 degrees F (175 degrees C).
2. Bring a pot of salted water to a boil. Cook pasta until flexible but not soft, about 5 minutes. Drain.
3. Heat oil in a stovetop- and oven-safe casserole dish over medium-high heat. Cook and stir chicken strips until browned, 3 to 5 minutes. Add onion, bell peppers, cherry tomatoes, olives, thyme, lemon zest, and pepper flakes. Cook and stir until the onions have begun to look translucent, about 5 minutes. Remove from heat. Stir in the half-cooked pasta.
4. Sprinkle Pecorino Romano and Grana Padano over the pasta mixture.
5. Bake in the preheated oven until bubbly and the cheeses have melted and browned, about 15 minutes. Let rest for 5 minutes before serving.

Mediterranean Chickpea Stew

PREPARATION
20 MIN

SERVES FOR
4 PEOPLE

INGREDIENTS

1/4 cup extra-virgin olive oil
1 large red onion, chopped
1 small bunch Italian parsley, minced
2 cloves garlic, minced
1 small carrot, coarsely shredded
1 small eggplant, cubed
2 cups cooked, sodium-free chickpeas, drained
1 cup cherry tomatoes, halved
1/2 cup vegetable broth, or more as needed
1 tablespoon dried oregano
1 teaspoon dried thyme
1/2 teaspoon cayenne pepper
salt and ground black pepper to taste

STEPS

1. Heat olive oil in a Dutch oven over medium heat. Add onion to the hot oil and cook until soft and translucent, about 5 minutes. Add parsley and garlic; cook and stir for 2 minutes. Add shredded carrot; stir often for 1 to 2 minutes. Add cubed eggplant and saute for 2 to 3 minutes.
2. Pour in chickpeas and tomatoes. Add broth, oregano, thyme, and cayenne pepper. Mix and bring to a boil. Reduce heat and simmer until stew has thickened and the vegetables are soft, about 15 minutes. Add more broth if necessary. Season with salt and pepper.

NUTRITION FACTS

Per Serving:

326 calories
protein 9.8g
carbohydrates 37g
fat 16.8g
sodium 124.9mg

Lebanese Lentil Soup (Shorbat Adas)

PREPARATION
25 MIN

SERVES FOR
4 PEOPLE

INGREDIENTS

2 tablespoons extra-virgin olive oil
1 onion, finely chopped
1 Yukon Gold potato, peeled and diced
1 carrot, peeled and diced
1 tomato, diced
2 celery ribs, diced
1 clove garlic, chopped, or more to taste
1 1/2 teaspoons kosher salt
3/4 teaspoon ground cumin
1/8 teaspoon ground cinnamon
1/8 teaspoon allspice
4 cups low-sodium vegetable broth
2 cups water
1 1/2 cups red lentils
2 lemons
2 pita bread, cut into squares
cooking spray
1 pinch salt

NUTRITION FACTS

Per Serving:

456 calories
protein 23.2g
carbohydrates 76.7g
fat 8.9g
sodium 1139.3mg

STEPS

1. Preheat the oven to 400 degrees F (200 degrees C).
2. Turn on a multi-functional pressure cooker and select Saute function. Heat olive oil in the pot. Add onion, potato, carrot, tomato, celery, and garlic; cook and stir until starting to soften, 3 to 5 minutes. Sprinkle salt, cumin, cinnamon, and allspice over the vegetables and stir until fragrant.
3. Pour in stock, water, and lentils. Close and lock the lid. Select high pressure according to manufacturer's instructions; set timer for 10 minutes. Allow 10 to 15 minutes for pressure to build.
4. Meanwhile, spread pita squares on a lined baking sheet. Spray with cooking spray and season with salt.
5. Bake in the preheated oven until toasted, about 8 minutes.
6. Release pressure carefully using the quick-release method according to manufacturer's instructions, about 5 minutes. Unlock and remove the lid. Puree soup using an immersion blender. Stir in juice of 1 lemon.
7. Divide soup among bowls and scatter a handful of pita chips over each. Cut the second lemon into wedges and serve alongside.

Pasta with Roasted Cauliflower and Parmesan

PREPARATION
20 MIN

SERVES FOR
8 PEOPLE

INGREDIENTS

1 medium head cauliflower, cut into bite-sized florets
5 cloves garlic, peeled and smashed
2 tablespoons olive oil, or more to taste
1/4 teaspoon salt
1/4 teaspoon ground black pepper
1 (16 ounce) package penne pasta
1 cup grated Parmesan cheese
1/4 cup seasoned bread crumbs
1 teaspoon ground cayenne pepper
2 tablespoons salted butter
1/4 cup lemon juice

STEPS

1. Preheat the oven to 425 degrees F (220 degrees C).
2. Toss cauliflower with garlic cloves, olive oil, salt, and pepper in a large bowl. Spread out in an even layer on a baking sheet.
3. Roast in the preheated oven, tossing at least twice, until cauliflower is tender, about 30 minutes.
4. Meanwhile, bring a large pot of lightly salted water to a boil. Add penne and cook, stirring occasionally, until tender yet firm to the bite, about 11 minutes.
5. Mix Parmesan cheese, bread crumbs, and cayenne pepper together in a bowl; set aside.
6. Drain pasta, reserving 1/2 cup cooking water. Transfer pasta to a serving bowl and add cauliflower and butter. Stir in cooking water, a little at a time, until desired creaminess is reached. Add lemon juice and bread crumb mixture, toss, and serve.

NUTRITION FACTS

Per Serving:

333 calories
protein 13.2g
carbohydrates 48.2g
fat 10.7g
cholesterol 16.5mg
sodium 332.4mg

CPSIA information can be obtained
at www.ICGtesting.com
Printed in the USA
BVHW051322140521
607268BV00006B/1476